Advance Praise for *Reset: An Introduction to Behavior Centered Design*

"Behavior Centered Design (BCD) is built on rich theory that most design approaches lack and practical global experience few practitioners have. The result is a flexible approach that can speak to digital or physical product design as well as to communication campaigns. Whether you are a seasoned behavior change expert or a newcomer, you will find refreshing depth in BCD."

—**Weston Baxter**, Professor of Design for Behavior Change,
Dyson School of Design, Imperial College

"A must read for any businesses seeking to make a positive difference to their consumers and societies in which they operate. It will provide the basis for genuinely integrating behavior change at the core of their business strategies. Full of great practical examples and framework to follow."

—**Myriam Sidibe**, Senior Fellow, Harvard Kennedy School and
author of *Brands on a Mission: How to Achieve
Social Impact and Business Growth through Purpose*

"A must-read for researchers, professionals, and policy makers! This book is an intellectual achievement and a milestone in the development of behavior change science. Behavior Centered Design stretches the limits of what we know about the mechanisms of behavior change and also provides a comprehensive and systematic theoretical framework to explain behavior change interventions in research, private and public sectors, and across contexts and populations."

—**Ivo Vlaev**, Professor of Behavioral Science,
University of Warwick Business School

Reset

An Introduction to Behavior Centered Design

ROBERT AUNGER

OXFORD
UNIVERSITY PRESS

OXFORD
UNIVERSITY PRESS

Oxford University Press is a department of the University of Oxford. It furthers
the University's objective of excellence in research, scholarship, and education
by publishing worldwide. Oxford is a registered trade mark of Oxford University
Press in the UK and certain other countries.

Published in the United States of America by Oxford University Press
198 Madison Avenue, New York, NY 10016, United States of America.

Library of Congress Cataloging-in-Publication Data
Names: Aunger, Robert, author.
Title: Reset : an introduction to behavior centered design / Robert Aunger.
Description: New York, NY : Oxford University Press, [2021] |
Includes bibliographical references and index.
Identifiers: LCCN 2020009319 (print) | LCCN 2020009320 (ebook) |
ISBN 9780197532638 (paperback) | ISBN 9780197532652 (epub) |
ISBN 9780197532669
Subjects: LCSH: Behavior modification.
Classification: LCC BF637.B4 A88 2021 (print) | LCC BF637.B4 (ebook) |
DDC 153.8/5—dc23
LC record available at https://lccn.loc.gov/2020009319
LC ebook record available at https://lccn.loc.gov/2020009320

9 8 7 6 5 4 3 2 1

Printed by LSC Communications, United States of America

CONTENTS

Preface vii

PART 1: Theory

1. What's the Problem? 3

2. Changing Behavior 19

3. Behavior Determination 31

PART 2: Practice

4. The Program Development Process 63

5. Assess 69

6. Build 81

7. Create 103

8. Deliver 111

9. Evaluate 117

10. What's Next? 125

Acknowledgments 135
Notes 137
References 141
Index 157

Why are professionals from a variety of fields becoming increasingly interested in behavior change? In public health, it's because we have failed to solve many of the world's most pressing health problems—and often not because we don't have solutions, but because they are not *used* enough. We know that stopping smoking, getting vaccinated, appropriate eating, safe sex, and exercise could solve the majority of the world's health problems, but they are simply not taken up sufficiently [1]. Similarly, marketers seek to make products more appealing to consumers but often don't know which insight would be key to changing consumers' buying habits. Their frustration is expressed in the famous quote (attributed to Henry Ford, among others): "I know half of our marketing efforts work; the problem is I don't know which half." Environmentalists eagerly point out the benefits of recycling and reducing our water use or carbon footprint, but we still fail to do these things. People also form intentions to change their own behavior (e.g., New Year's resolutions and dieting plans) but often fail to follow through. All of these situations require a better understanding of how to change human behavior.

Until recently, most approaches to behavior change have been based in trying to change individual cognition in one way or another, either by changing the way people consciously appraise their experiences [2–4] or modifying cognitive rules of thumb for making judgments (called *heuristics*)—the techniques used by behavioral economists [5, 6]. Opportunity, Ability, and Motivation (OAM) approaches are also popular but are based on models of persuasive communication. That is, they are basically designed to produce changes to attitudes, rather than behavior change [7–10]. Few approaches are firmly based on the latest thinking about human behavior itself, the purposes that it evolved to serve, or the way in which it changes in response to changing environmental circumstances. People largely *know* what they should be doing—being more active, not smoking, getting regular medical check-ups—but just don't *do* them. So behavior change programs need to focus on **behavior** and its real-world context, not just on human cognition or communication. With the recent revolutions in our understanding of situations [11–13], environments [14], and brains [15], it is time to update our approach to behavior change.

Behavior Centered Design (BCD) is a new framework that aims to embody these recent advances [16]. As the name implies, it is centered on behavior. It begins with the insight that the need for change arises when normal learning from behavior fails (because learning will normally take care of maladaptive patterns of behavior). It provides a coherent behavioral model derived from reinforcement learning theory, develops a fundamental taxonomy of needs based in evolutionary biology, shows how the disruption of environmental settings is key, and sets out the steps involved in programming for behavior change. So, as well as providing a means of identifying the levers that can change behavior, it also provides a design process, with steps and tools to use in conceiving, creating, implementing, and evaluating a behavior change program. This approach mixes both science *and* creativity because behavior will only change in response to something new and challenging [17–19]. The approach has been employed successfully on a range of public health behaviors as well as in commercial product design and marketing.

This book is designed to encourage behavior change practitioners to think differently about behavior—both in understanding how and why it is produced and in how to design programs to change it. It is broken into two parts, concerned with theory and practice, respectively. *Reset* begins in Part 1 with an in-depth presentation of the theory behind BCD. How BCD conceptualizes the behavior change challenge is first taken up. Unlike traditional approaches that start and end with changing cognitions, I emphasize other factors—and include the key principles of *Surprise, Revaluation*, and *Performance*. In Chapter 3, I provide a list of all the things that can influence behavior, as a way of ensuring that no stone is left unturned when formulating a behavior change strategy. Part 2 is a manual for how to develop a behavior change program, step by step—from *Assess* through to *Evaluate*—using tools and procedures developed by those who have been associated with the BCD approach. I provide many examples along the way, as well as further material, which I encourage you to consult via the links and suggested literature. However, it begins with a short introduction to the BCD approach, describing its main contentions, with a summary of the BCD process of program development (for those who may have skipped the theoretical Part 1).

Whether you take just some elements from BCD or use it throughout to design a program, it should help you to find creative ways of changing behavior that are surprising, that add value, and that improve the performance of the people in your program. In this way, I hope it can help to make the world a place where more people can flourish.

Reset

Theory

This book is broken into two major parts, on Theory and Practice. Given the complexities of behavior determination, it is important to rely on theory, at least implicitly, to effectively modify behavior. Part 1 therefore presents an introduction to the theoretical resources that inform Behavior Centered Design (BCD), the approach that forms the focus of this book. Theory from evolutionary biology and psychology will be covered and then organized around the problem of behavior change.

Part 2 concerns the process of designing behavior change programs (which can concern a single individual trying to help themselves to a change in their own behavior, or an entire population). The BCD approach to program development bears considerable similarity to program design processes in various fields, although it does emphasize the importance of focusing on the observation of actual situations (to better "reset" them) and creativity in dealing with the opportunities and barriers uncovered. It therefore makes use of a number of tools that have been designed to facilitate uncovering these barriers and opportunities more effectively, which are presented at appropriate junctures in the process description.

What's the Problem?

Behavior change has recently come to be recognized as an important objective in many fields:

- Public policy (to increase compliance with governmental initiatives)
- Marketing (to achieve brand switching or brand loyalty)
- Education (to improve student outcomes)
- Business management (to increase profits)
- Health promotion (to achieve public health improvements)
- City planning (to advance the design of buildings and public spaces)
- Sport psychology (to improve performance)
- Website design (to improve the user experience)
- Self-help efforts (e.g., financial goal achievement).

It is being heralded as a policy cure-all in the halls of government, as the latest fad to improve learning in schools or to make marketing more scientific, and as a necessary lynchpin of successful programs in public health. Behavior change is thus a hot topic in many fields.

The concept of behavior change implies that preferred courses of action are perceived as possible but tend not to occur. It is often seen as being hard to achieve. Failed New Year's resolutions, neglected dieting regimes, and unused gym subscriptions are given as examples. However, changes in behavior are happening everywhere, all the time. Social life has changed considerably: we now live in megalopolises and fly from continent to continent. Some people now cope with multiple switches in their jobs over their career (whereas people used to be born and die in the same profession, and previous to that, everyone had the same profession: farmer!). We participate in numerous social networks (e.g., church members, bridge club, work groups, sports teams, hobby clubs) rather than just being kin or neighbors. People have learned to deal with novel institutions: children spend half their daily lives in school; many people now keep some of their money in a bank and use "virtual money" in the form of credit cards or bitcoin. People take regular baths, give birth in hospitals, drive cars, wear glasses or hearing aids, take a pill to prevent conceptions, and fling dirty dishes into a dishwasher.

In 1985, no one could telephone others while they were "on the run"; 30 years later, many people in the poorest villages in the developing world are using mobile phones. The Internet has disrupted many old behaviors since its introduction around 1995: interpersonal communication (letter-writing to email to Twitter), consumption patterns (physical to online shopping), and even reading books (now done on screens rather than in printed form). In fact, for this increasingly important kind of behavior change—learning to live with new technologies—the rate of adoption is becoming *faster* with time: mobile phones have become endemic in only a few years, whereas regular showering took many years to become popular (http://www.karlhartig.com/chart/techhouse.pdf). So, in many ways, human psychology is exquisitely tuned to producing the most appropriate response to what a changing environment throws up. The rate at which populations change their behavior is actually increasing, along with the rate of technological advancement.

This is possible because human behavior is highly flexible; it responds rapidly to changes in the environment. Not all organisms can do this; those that can't respond to rapid environmental changes or have a narrow diet or niche may go extinct as a result [20]. Even complex behaviors can be programmed by genes if the environment remains stable long enough. However, in stochastic environments, the optimal course of action can change more rapidly than genetic changes can track. Further, if many tasks must be achieved through behavior, competition and conflict can arise between goals, requiring contextualized switching between tasks, which also means the optimal course of behavior at a given moment can be different. So, species such as animals that depend on behavior for solving many tasks can also run into complex decision-making problems.

Producing adaptive behavior in complex or stochastic environments thus requires considerable mental agility. Animals in general have had to succeed under conditions that require a high degree of flexibility, as their environments tend to fluctuate rapidly [21–23]. The ability to reliably produce quick, responsive kinds of interaction with stochastic environments was enabled in animals by the development of a nervous system, which had the ability to detect and classify the animal's situation, as well as to store information that could be of benefit in selecting appropriate responses when encountering similar conditions later—that is, they evolved the ability to learn from experience [16, 24, 25]. The nervous system is able, first, to direct complex movements of various body parts relatively quickly and, second, to store information acquired through feedback from behavioral choices in the form of memory. Complex behavior—such as humans exhibit—thus has the purpose of keeping bodies alive and reproducing through rapid, flexible self-propelled bodily movement, producing a functional interaction between the animal and its environment [26–28]. It is the combination of rapid behavioral learning, in response to environmental changes, enabled by nervous systems, that characterizes the animal mega-adaptation.

Human evolution has been characterized by particularly violent and shifting selection pressures, as a result of environmental fluctuations, particularly over the last 10,000 years [29, 30]. This history has left its mark in terms of a large brain for coping with these rapid changes. Indeed, we can be said to have evolved particularly large brains to cope with recurrent and rapid environmental variability during our evolution [31]. Further, as previously discussed, environmental changes have only increased in speed with more recent technological developments. So, we are becoming more and more reliant on producing adaptively plastic or flexible responses to changing environmental conditions as time goes on.

This evolutionary perspective suggests that if there is a need to change behavioral responses to particular situations, it must be due to some inability to adapt appropriately to environmental change through the usual evolutionary mechanisms. Indeed, I will argue that *the need to change behavior overtly has typically arisen because environmental conditions exist that prohibit effective learning and hence performance of the appropriate behavioral choice.* I will show in the following discussion that, under certain conditions, learning does not work adaptively, so that particular kinds of discrepancies can arise between what the environment throws up and how psychological mechanisms can gain knowledge from experience of those situations. Further, those situations tend to be the ones in which people nowadays seek to induce changes in behavior—either in themselves or others.

BCD is a new and radically different approach to the problem of changing behavior that begins with the insight that behavior change is an adaptive learning problem [16]. It recognizes that the primary challenge is to overcome some hurtle to effectively learn the appropriate response to a situation and then implement it. Using an evolutionary framework, BCD unites the latest findings about how brains learn with a practical set of steps and tools to design successful behavior change programs. (Here, I typically assume interest in relatively large-scale programs; however, I also present scenarios illustrating how BCD can be applied in more individualized behavior change contexts, such as self-help and changing the minds of policymakers, later in the book.) In the rest of this chapter, I first outline how learning normally works and then detail how it might go wrong, setting up the conditions for a need to intervene.

HOW LEARNING WORKS

To better understand how learning can fail to happen appropriately, I first model how learning is supposed to work, so that I can pinpoint the ways in which the system can break down.

Making optimal choices about how to behave can be a difficult proposition, partly because of the "credit assignment problem" [32]: outcomes in complex situations may depend on a series of actions, only the last of which provides a reward or punishment. This means that feedback can be delayed, and it can be difficult to determine where the decision-making process went wrong. Think of a chess game in which you play for 50 moves and then lose. How can you learn which move doomed you to failure in the end—the 3rd move, the 23rd, or the 43rd?

Reinforcement learning (RL) is an algorithm that can solve this problem [33]. Although originally developed in computer science to study machine learning and the optimum control of production processes, it has also been widely used in psychology and neuroscience. RL is currently the best-established computational model of how autonomous agents such as animals and robots acquire information through experience with their environment. Indeed, RL has been independently validated, using different kinds of criteria and standards of practice, in four very different fields: control theory/operations research, artificial intelligence/machine learning, neuroscience, and psychology [34]. The RL-based way of modeling the predictive brain has thus become the dominant approach to understanding neuroscientific processes [35, 36] in modeling human learning from behavior [37], intelligent robot behavior production [38, 39], and operations management [33]. This is because it has been found that the brain's reward system operates in a fashion consistent with the mathematical formalizations of RL [40], because robots programmed with software that operates using RL algorithms produce the most sophisticated behavior [41] and because using the RL formalism produces a very efficient and effective means of describing organizational changes generally [42]. For example, a computer-based software agent using RL can play computer games at human expert level [43]. RL is also being used to develop robots that can explore unknown territories while minimizing collisions with obstacles [44].

More specifically, the RL mechanism has now been shown to characterize motivated learning in brains, in which there is a close correspondence between the behavior of mesolimbic dopaminergic neurons and the prediction error term described in formal temporal difference models of RL [45]. This correspond-ence has been demonstrated both in monkeys [46, 47] and humans [48–50]. Such neuronal signaling can be used to revise expectations from experience and to learn new behaviors [51]. So, evidence is accumulating that the mechanisms hypothesized by this computational model characterize the way human brains actually work [35].

RL is designed to describe the everyday processes by which robots or people learn, via trial and error, to act upon a changing environment so as to maximize a future stream of rewards, based on only partial knowledge of their world. RL explains how such agents can adapt their behavior to varying contingencies by repeatedly updating their estimates of the rewarding value of alternative actions, thanks to feedback received from the environment as a consequence of their action. This can lead, over time, to different responses to the same stimulus—behavior change. Thus, RL suggests that learning is about correcting errors [52]. Hence, if learning fails, errors persist—potentially requiring an intervention to change behavior.

Indeed, one can see the brain as essentially a machine for making predictions about what will happen in the world if one perturbs it (through behavior) in some way [15]. From this perspective, the person's job is to identify a policy that maps perceived states of the world to actions that maximizes some measure of long-term reinforcement (as an indicator of having done "the right thing"). Reinforcement signals can be computed at various points during the time over which a goal is being pursued. Learning occurs whenever there are discrepancies between the level of reward that is expected from a behavior and that which is actually received after it has been executed. A temporal difference error alerts the psychological system to situations in which the change in value of the current state from the previous state (brought about through behavior) is significantly different from what was expected—that is, when there hasn't been as much progress toward achievement of the goal as should have occurred by this point [33, 53]. This allows the brain to adjust expected levels of reward during the process of goal pursuit and, hence, produce adaptive responses to changing circumstances [54].

The model adopted here to understand the psychological foundations of behavior change—which embodies a version of RL—can be seen in Figure 1.1 (based on Figure 1 from Singh et al. [55]).[1] This representation can be thought of as two causal loops—since the brain lies within body and the body, within the environment—but is presented as spatially independent loops for pictorial clarity (an embedded version is presented in a later chapter).

The basic RL model has been augmented to make it more realistic in ecological terms. This is necessary as the RL literature was originally purely computational (or information-theoretic) in nature. In particular, the body is given physical reality by adding physiological processes of metabolism and arousal, while the environment is allowed to provide the body with resources such as food and social companionship. The environment is also granted endogenous responses because it includes other agents, such as animals as well as other humans, and so will respond adaptively to behavioral stimulation by the focal individual. Further, the brain also responds to rewards and perceived changes to the environment by updating its model of the world (learning) and storing this information for later use (memory).[2]

I can now describe the subprocesses that take place during an instance of RL in greater detail. According to the model, a causal cycle begins in the brain, and,

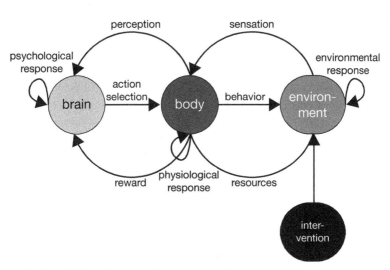

Figure 1.1. The BCD reinforcement learning model.
Source: Based on Singh et al. [55].

based on current knowledge of the state of the world, an animal or robot uses the RL algorithm to compute the value expected from various behavioral options. Based on these values, an action selection process picks the highest valued option and instructs the motor cortex to perform the selected action sequence, which is stored (for future use) as the optimal option for that situation. These instructions cause a metabolic response and arousal in the body that produces a behavior or interaction between the body and its environment [14]. Behavior results in a change to the state of the environment (e.g., chasing a prey causes a change in location of one's body in relation to the physical surroundings), which can cause endogenous reactions by the environment (e.g., a prey avoids capture by engaging in independent movement). The consequences of behavior are thus a combination of the activity of the body and the environmental response. This outcome is what is sensed by the body (e.g., the prey is seen running away) as the first sort of feedback. Resources can also be acquired through the behavior (e.g., meat through capture of the prey). Consumption or use of the resources provides changes to the peripheral nervous system, transmitted to the brain, which converts the sensations from the peripheral nervous system into perceptions of changes in the environment and the body's internal states. On this basis, the brain calculates a reward as the information from perception and resources acquired minus the metabolic/arousal costs of producing the behavior in the first place. Rewards are subjective, or psychological—positive if the action resulted in an environmental change consistent with the animal's goal (e.g., chasing a prey resulted in the prey being captured) or negative if not. Learning and memory then take place as endogenous changes in the brain. The brain allows the animal to associate the perceived changes produced in the environment by the behavior with the resulting reward (positive or negative) from prior action selection—an instance of RL. Learning is the changes in the brain due to this reward and perceptual processing (i.e., an association of reward to prior action selection and perception of the environmental response). Memory storage can be another consequence of the psychological response.

Note that the process runs repeatedly; that is, after learning is complete, in the next time frame, the cycle begins anew, with the animal selecting another action, given the new state of the environment, and getting feedback in the form of a reward and perception of new changes in the environment, resulting from the new behavior. Thanks to RL, actions that lead to positive rewards tend to be repeated when similar circumstances present themselves again. Over time, the animal learns to perform actions that tend to result in high payoffs—as expected if behavior is an adaptation to produce effective responses to a variety of environmental conditions. Indeed, robots programmed with RL algorithms come to perform behavioral patterns consistent with expectations from evolutionary theories about behavior. For example, teams of robots using different strategies allocate their energy in "food quests" in ways consistent with competition between species in the same niche from optimal foraging theory [57].

Essentially, the RL perspective suggests that the brain's expectations should be consistent with what the world is likely to actually offer, because thinking unrealistically would likely lead to dangers or lost opportunities. Thus, what an animal requires is to have the most accurate mirror of the real world in its brain that it is feasible to produce, given constraints on experience and information-processing capabilities.

The model also includes the possibility of an intervention as the primary means of inducing behavior change. An intervention is typically a form of behavior by an outside party (e.g., a message spoken to a friend, a billboard on the side of a bus), but this behavior may have already occurred (e.g., in the form of an environmental modification with which the target behavior will interact), only be planned (with the intention to see how the intervention will influence other model elements), or be unnecessary (as in the case of a self-induced decision to lose weight through a self-help program); hence, the link is represented as a dotted line in the model (Figure 1.1).

With its concentration on feedback loops between the brain, body, and environment and the possibility of interjecting some novel element into the cycle, the BCD RL model has structural similarities to the existing approaches to behavior change: Social Regulation Theory [58], the Antecedent–Behavior–Consequence (or ABC) model used in Applied Behavioral Analysis [59], and the Transtheoretical approach [60]. They are all composed of positive feedback loops (e.g., between Antecedents, Behavior, and Consequences in the case of the ABC approach or Inputs, Throughput, and Output in the Self-Regulation Model). In effect, no model of change (as opposed to behavior determination) has been developed that doesn't involve an intervention at some point in the body-environmental interaction—a modification that, once induced, feeds forward to the other model components. This suggests that there is something fundamental about seeing change in cyclical terms—a point with which the BCD approach is consistent.

Learning is not the only brain function that has been characterized as using error correction as a mechanism. Error correction has also been demonstrated to characterize perception (as minimization of prediction coding) [61], action selection (as the neuroeconomic principle to maximize expected utility) [62], memory (as world-model updating to minimize surprisal) [63], and motor control (as forward modeling to minimize the discrepancy between expected and perceived body position) [64]. As a result, there is a growing consensus that error correction should be recognized as a mechanism characteristic of the brain's operation as a whole. Authors reaching this conclusion have called this perspective the Bayesian brain [65], the predictive brain [66], and the proactive brain [67] and the global mechanism itself, the free energy principle [68], failure modes [69], and nested intelligence [70]. I will refer to RL and its generalization, the predictive brain hypothesis, interchangeably here.

Only a few behaviors do not participate in the normal error correction-based learning process, but these are the ones that everyone focuses on, as they cause problems or are otherwise less than optimal from some perspective (e.g., produce insufficient sales or market share). The behavior change problem is therefore one of overcoming learning difficulties. The BCD approach (introduced more formally in Part 2 of this book) is the result of an effort to design an approach to behavior change that takes its inspiration directly from this insight—because that should more reliably lead to appropriate solutions and, hence, more effective interventions. From this perspective, the problem is that *some* behaviors are *persistently resistant* to change. People know they should do their homework, clean house, save money for retirement, quit smoking, eat healthier diets, and exercise more but find it difficult to actually do so. Typically these behaviors affect large groups of people and so become problematic—both at an individual and public level. It is only in these few cases that behavior has "gone wrong" and can't be modified effectively. So behavior change isn't hard per se; it's only hard when you notice there's a problem because the desired change isn't happening.

WAYS LEARNING CAN GO WRONG

Overcoming error correction failures requires knowing what kinds of failures can arise. I will now look to see exactly what kinds of learning failures can be associated with the need to change behavior and whether the BCD approach, founded on RL, can account for them. I will take the field of public health as our field of inquiry because an obvious consequence of maladaptation is a failure to thrive, and public health is charged with understanding the causes of widespread morbidity and mortality. This field should therefore have good evidence of the kinds of maladaptation that can arise and cause the kinds of problems that people want to ameliorate through behavior change.

Public health officials measure morbidity and mortality costs in terms of disability-adjusted life-years (DALYs). If we look at the top 20 risk factors associated with lost DALYs on the global scale today, we see that each factor can be associated with both novel technologies and particular behaviors (Table 1.1). For example, obesity (or overweight) as a medical condition is associated with a variety of common "diseases of civilization" such as cardiovascular disease and diabetes, as well as the availability of industrial foods with artificially high concentrations of fat and salt, coupled with the advent of domestic labor-saving devices such as washing machines and dishwashers. The behavioral consequences are overconsumption of calories and increased sedentarism, which lead to an imbalance between energy intake and expenditure. Similar stories can be told for each of the other major causes of lost DALYs.

It is not surprising to find that specific behaviors underlie these problems— hence the recognition that behavior change is important in the public health field. What is more surprising is the involvement of novel technologies such as refined foods, cigarettes, condoms, and cars, either as an aspect of the problem or as part of the solution for each major disease risk.

The involvement of technology becomes more understandable when it is realized that technological innovation can occur many times within a generation, while the brains of individuals—that have to learn to engage with new technologies— are produced by genes, which are modified only once per demographic generation

Table 1.1. Top 20 Global Causes of Lost DALYs

Risk Factor for Burden of Disease	Health Outcomes	Contributory Causes to Risk Factors	Novel Technologies	Novel Behaviors
1. Underweight	Malnutrition, infection, low birthweight	Economic factors, industrialization and mass production of food	Detrimental: convenience foods	Loss of traditional feeding practices (e.g., bottle feeding, weaning)
2. Unsafe sex	STDs (HIV), cervical cancer	Rural–urban migration, social breakdown, sex industry, cultural factors	Beneficial: condoms	Increased same/opposite sex promiscuity
3. High blood pressure	Cardiovascular disease, stroke	Industrialization and mass production of food, sedentarization of work and leisure	Detrimental: refined salt, sugar, oils, etc. Labor-saving and leisure technologies	Overconsumption, sedentary lifestyle
4. Tobacco	Cancer, heart disease, respiratory disease	Industrialization and mass production of cheap psychoactive drug	Detrimental: tobacco high in available nicotine (cigarettes)	Smoking
5. Alcohol	Cancer, heart disease, diabetes, depression, injuries	Industrialization and mass production of cheap psychoactive drug	Detrimental: refined alcoholic drinks	Regular and binge drinking
6. Water, sanitation and hygiene	Diarrheal disease, respiratory infection	Insufficient public/private investment in water supply and sanitation	Beneficial: soap, toilet, water treatment devices	Handwashing, toilet and water filter use
7. High cholesterol	Cardiovascular disease, stroke	Industrialization and mass production of processed foods, sedentarization of work and leisure	Detrimental: low-density lipoproteins and trans fats	Use of processed foods, sedentary lifestyle
8. Indoor smoke	Respiratory disease	Cooking with solid fuels, house design	Beneficial: improved stoves	Use of solid fuels for cooking
9. Iron deficiency	Anemia, malnutrition, infection	Cereal-based diets, recurrent infection, helminth infection, early weaning	Beneficial: micronutrient supplements	Consumption of cereals/weaning foods

(continued)

Table 1.1. CONTINUED

Risk Factor for Burden of Disease	Health Outcomes	Contributory Causes to Risk Factors	Novel Technologies	Novel Behaviors
10. Overweight	Cardiovascular disease, stroke, diabetes, cancer	Industrialization and mass production of processed foods, sedentarization of work and leisure	Detrimental: refined salt/sugar/oils, labor-saving and leisure technologies	Over-consumption, sedentary lifestyle
11. Zinc deficiency	Anemia, malnutrition, infection	Cereal-based diets, recurrent infection, helminth infection, early weaning	Beneficial: micronutrient supplements	Consumption of cereals/weaning foods
12. Low fruit and vegetable intake	Cardiovascular disease, stroke, cancer	Industrialization, mass production of processed foods	Detrimental: refined salt/sugar/oils	Consumption of processed foods
13. Vitamin A deficiency	Anemia, malnutrition, infection	Cereal-based diets, recurrent infection, helminth infection, early weaning	Beneficial: micronutrient supplements	Consumption of cereals/weaning foods
14. Physical inactivity	Cardiovascular disease, stroke, cancer	Sedentarization of work and leisure	Detrimental: labor-saving and leisure technologies	Sedentary lifestyle
15. Occupational	Injury	Industrialization	Detrimental: industrial machinery	Interaction with machinery
16. Lead exposure	Cardiovascular disease, mental retardation	Industrialization, mass production of automated transportation	Detrimental: cars, lorries	Driving
17. Illicit drug use	HIV, overdose, injury, infection	Production and marketing of cheap psychoactive drugs	Detrimental: refined psychoactive compounds, syringes	Drug consumption/injection
18. Unsafe injections	Acute infection	Contaminated injections	Detrimental: syringes	Syringe reuse
19. Lack of contraception	Maternal mortality	Cultural factors, lack of access	Beneficial: contraceptive technologies	Uptake of contraception
20. Childhood sexual abuse	Depression, alcohol abuse	Cultural factors		

Original from Ezzati, M., Hoorn, S., Rodgers, A., Lopez, A., Mathers, C., Murray, C., & Group, C. R. A. C. (2003). Estimates of global and regional potential health gains from reducing multiple major risk factors. *Lancet, 362*, 271–280, as adapted and augmented by Curtis, V., & Aunger, R. (2011). Motivational mismatch: Evolved motives as the source of—and solution to—global public health problems. In S. C. Roberts (Ed.), *Applied Evolutionary Psychology* (pp. 259–275). Oxford: Oxford University Press.

(about 25 years in humans). Since the Pleistocene, the rate of technological innovation has increased over time. So, whereas it took nearly a million years for primitive hand-axes to become more sophisticated, it now requires only a few years for new versions of popular devices like computers or cars to be produced. Thus, techno-generations have become shorter in many cases than demographic generations. As a result, technological evolution often proceeds more rapidly than genetic evolution, leading to a mismatch between what brains suggest is an appropriate behavioral response to some environmental stimulus and what would actually be appropriate in the techno-environments created by human groups [1]. So environmental conditions can change too rapidly for evolved psychological mechanisms such as RL to cope effectively.

Can RL deficits really account for public health problems in a systematic and theoretically sound way? In the family of RL models, there can be two kinds of error, each associated with one of the two pathways from the body to the brain in the BCD RL model (Figure 1.1) [71]. The first one is about the nature of what is perceived (i.e., some situational incongruity about the state of the environment, such as seeing snow on a tropical beach). This kind of error is called *perceptual* because it is based on a state prediction error about the state of the world. It constitutes the Surprise stream in the Figure 1.1, which begins at the top of the diagram with novel sensations, culminating in a psychological response.

The second cause, *utility surprise*, is about the value of the environmental response to the animal (in terms of whether it is likely to satisfy some need), which has proved higher or lower than expected. This is called a *reward prediction error*, which is associated with the Revaluation stream in Figure 1.1. It works its way up from the bottom of the diagram with resources being provided as feedback from behavior, which spawns a reward calculation.

We can be even more specific about the kinds of mismatch between technological and psychological processes that account for major public health problems by noting that there are four kinds of pathological process, or conditions under which normal learning does not take place, so that the problems persist without being rectified through experience (Table 1.2). Two of these conditions involve state prediction errors, and two, reward prediction errors.

The first kind of state prediction error arises when a novel technology is highly motivating when properly used but nevertheless doesn't provide evolutionary benefits. These tend to be bio-technologies that are intrinsically rewarding (because they mimic the brain's own reward system), which were designed to be stimulating and, hence, get widely used to excess, such as synthetically produced alcohol and tobacco (DALY risks #4 and #5 in the list from Table 1.1). Smoking and drinking mimic the effects of goal achievement without the normal pairing of some form of adaptive behavior. Hence, the behavior can be considered nonfunctional, as it doesn't produce any resources. Instead, a drug is simply ingested, but it provides the same effects as achieving a real goal—and directly to the brain (which reinforces an "easy" route to reward and hence stimulates further drug-taking and often physiological addiction as well). Thus, the *Reward Mimic problem* is that a technology (drugs) produces rewards that simulate the brain's dopamine-based

Table 1.2. TYPES OF PATHOLOGICAL LEARNING

Case	Problem	Top 20 Risk Factor Examples	Solutions
State prediction errors			
Reward mimic	Rewarding object use is not associated with evolutionary goal achievement.	Tobacco, alcohol and psychoactive drugs	Interrupt reward pathway; substitute alternative rewarding behavior.
Super stimulating	Object use is more rewarding than expected	Salt, fat and carbohydrate-dense foods	Add punishments to use.
Reward prediction errors			
Side effect	Everyday experience doesn't include rare punishments.	Labor-saving means of production/ transport; syringe reuse; environmental toxins as by-product of industrial production; lead poisoning	Emphasize potential punishments.
Temporal imbalance	Distant rewards are offset by current punishments.	Convenience foods, micronutrient supplements, sanitation, soap, condoms, cooking stoves.	Increase expected value from object use; improve object so it becomes more rewarding

reward system without providing any of the benefits normally associated with goal achievement.

Another problem is that humans have difficulty controlling their intake of technologically enhanced "natural" goods such as foods because they are super stimulating. With *Super Stimulation*, a given level of consumption results in the overproduction of benefits. In the case of food consumption, there is unwanted fat production, for example, due to the unnatural calorie and nutrient densities of manufactured foods. The trick that arises here is a surprising level of reward in return for a particular behavior (e.g., consumption of a certain amount of food).

Then there are two kinds of reward prediction error scenarios. The first of these involves novel technologies that are rewarding for the vast majority of the time but that can occasionally have harmful *Side Effects*. Driving is an example. Automobiles are an excellent way of getting quickly from point A to point B, but because the current infrastructure causes people going from point B to point A to drive right alongside those going in the opposite direction, there are sometimes deadly collisions, essentially as a side effect of the speed that cars enable people to move across the landscape. Thus, use of automobiles in over 99% of trips is rewarding but in rare cases (not often experienced by a given individual) can be significantly punishing (e.g., via an accident). However, this pattern of use teaches the evolved learning system that cars are such a "good thing" that precautions (such as wearing seatbelts) do not seem necessary.

Another example from the list of top 20 morbidity causes is domestic appliances that increase productivity but when used in combination and without other compensation can reduce physical activity to such a degree that obesity results (risk #10, as previously discussed). So, the Side-Effect learning pathology can involve incidental, infrequent consequences of a regular behavior, but since such consequences do not always accompany the behavior, they are not part of the normal learning process associated with its performance. Alternatively, the punishments (e.g., an accident while driving) are not as strong as the typical (functional) outcome (e.g., reduced travel times) and so do not overwhelm the positive rewards and therefore do not eliminate the practice.

Second, the use of some novel health-giving technologies may not be intrinsically motivating, or at least not sufficiently rewarding to inspire use (given the costs of use, perhaps), or are rewarding in ways that don't lead to appropriate use (e.g., at the wrong time). For example, techno-evolution has thrown up some new technologies that help alleviate various disease conditions, such as condoms to prevent the spread of sexually transmitted diseases like HIV (risk #2). However, because they are perceived to reduce sexual pleasure, condoms tend to be ignored. Effectively, the problem is a *Temporal Imbalance (of rewards)*, which makes this technology a failed solution to a problem: people are still dying when they need not, given existing technology (if only people would use it).[3] In Temporal Imbalance, the normal reward associated with performance of the target behavior (with the appropriate technological aid) is negative (reduced sexual pleasure) but is accompanied by long-term benefits (avoidance of sexually transmitted diseases and hence enjoy a longer life). However, the discounting of these future benefits cannot compensate for the immediate punishments. Hence, the learning process leads to avoidance of the healthy behavior. Learning is occurring appropriately in this case; it is just that the technological aid does not have a pattern of reward for use that is net reinforcing.[4]

In sum, Reward-Mimicking technologies use the body (e.g., via signals that stimulate dopamine) to trick the brain; Super-Stimulating technologies fool the brain into thinking that use of objects is not as rewarding as it really is. Temporal Imbalance is due to an object not providing sufficient stimulation during use but is coupled with long-term benefits. Finally, Side-Effect mismatch is due to the brain being unable to calculate the appropriate reward function, given the structure of experience. In each of these scenarios, the RL feedback process is disrupted in some way. Each of these problems "tricks" the learning system in a way that precludes effective learning.

MISMATCH-SPECIFIC SOLUTIONS

How can the BCD approach, using the lens of RL, help elucidate—and, potentially, ameliorate—the psychological mismatch that appears to lie at the center of most behavior change problems? The suggestion is that the intervention should be designed to overcome the type of mismatch that is at the root of the problem. This is certainly true in the domain of public health.

Reward mimics are difficult to combat. One possibility would be to *interrupt or eliminate the reward pathway* (e.g., chemically). For example, electronic cigarettes imitate the feeling of inhaling smoke using a safer vapor lacking in nicotine. Alternatively, one could *substitute an alternative, equally rewarding behavior*. This too can be difficult but sometimes works. For example, some people chew gum every time they feel the desire to smoke.

Solutions in this case can resort to legislation as well, because such problems can't be reliably motivated at an individual level. For example, smoking and alcohol consumption are highly regulated (who can buy, who can sell, where consumption is allowed). This category of mismatch often has to deal with the physiological dependencies that can arise from prolonged use. For smoking, this can be done through nicotine patches or similar methods to resolve nicotine dependency; alternatively, supportive social environments can be provided for those who wish to quit cold turkey (e.g., rehabilitation hostels).

Like Reward Mimics, Super-Stimulating mismatch behaviors must be stopped or downregulated, not started or upregulated. *Adding punishments* to the use of Super-Stimulating objects is the primary mechanism here. This can be achieved, for example, through social stigmatization (e.g., eating super-calorific fast food products may be cast as "low class"). Price disincentives can be brought to bear as well (e.g., high taxation on cigarettes and alcohol)—at least where the option of legislation is likely to be effective down to the individual level, thanks to good governance (e.g., in modern democracies).

The obvious strategy for Side-Effect problems is to *emphasize the potential negative consequences of behavioral practice*. For example, driving-speed reduction campaigns often make graphic presentations of traffic accidents (e.g., the bodies of loved ones flying out of cars or dead by the roadside). These campaigns attempt to "make real" the worst consequences of the behavior. However, public health workers often find it difficult to curb behavior at an individual level, so outside pressures can be brought to bear—hence, the prevalence of legislative solutions for this kind of mismatch (e.g., seat belts and airbags are required components of car manufacturing processes; who can buy and sell guns or injection needles is severely regulated). Of course, mandating provision of seat belts does not guarantee their use.

Programs stymied by Temporal Imbalance mismatch have the problem of increasing the use of a novel technological solution. For example, hygiene problems are often due to lack of uptake (e.g., of soap for handwashing, toothpaste for toothbrushing, or surface cleaner for household surfaces), because such products are only minimally rewarding to use. One way in which uptake can be increased is by *adding value to use of the unrewarding object*—a typical job performed by marketing efforts for new products (e.g., by making them "sexy" or "cool"). Alternatively, the technological solution can itself be *improved so that it is more rewarding* (e.g., like good-smelling, nonabrasive soap).

With this argument, I have shown that the BCD approach is able not only to identify the most important factors underlying problem behaviors but can also explain *why* certain behaviors become persistent public health problems in the first place: a small set of pathological learning processes an important cause of most of the most severe public health problems at a global scale (although additional sorts of pathological learning may exist and characterize other behavior change fields, such as education or policy).[5]

It is interesting to note that each major risk factor thus has the inappropriate use of some novel technology as an important cause or the appropriate use of a novel technology as a way of eliminating or avoiding that disease. In effect, *novel technologies are either the source of each problem or part of its solution.* (This doesn't mean that some change in technology is always going to be the intervention in a behavior change campaign or program, just that technology frames the issue the campaign seeks to address in the first place.) What this analysis suggests is that behavior change interventions should modify what these behavioral problems have in common: undesirable forms of learning from interaction with a novel technology.

Similar kinds of mismatch are likely to characterize other areas where behavior change is required (e.g., policy, marketing, self-help), so I suggest that this is probably a general finding. In Temporal Imbalance cases, for example, the public health strategy is to *increase the expected value of performance.* Adding value to use of a product is a standard marketing challenge and can be done by associating a brand with new kinds of rewards. Public health programs can do the same thing, using the same "tricks." Similarly, from a marketing perspective, the aim of a company is typically to increase sales or the market share of a product, which implies that *more* of the product should be used or consumed. Due to the high level of reward associated with product use, these products "sell themselves," so the psychological challenge becomes one of branding—getting consumers to prefer the company's own version of the product. Thus, we get the Coke versus Pepsi wars and the Apple versus Samsung mobile phone battles.

However, the interests of public health government, and commercial enterprises can also differ with respect to a given kind of learning failure. For example, I have said that Side-Effect mismatch in public health requires emphasizing the potential downsides of use, such as car accidents. Car manufacturer advertisements, on the other hand, will often suggest their products are very safe and that no harm will come to the driver even if there is an accident (although even more often, they won't mention the problem, preferring to leave it forgotten, thanks to its rarity). So which behavior change challenge arises from a given type of learning failure can depend on the aim of the program, which can differ as a function of stakeholder interest.

The BCD approach suggests that behavior change efforts should be clear about how the target behavior in a given project fails to be subject to adaptive learning. That is, it must classify the learning disability that lies at the heart of the problem (see Table 1.2). Program managers should also determine how the proposed intervention will clear the learning blockage. How BCD tackles this job is described in the next chapter.

2

Changing Behavior

I have identified reinforcement learning failures as central to situations in which behavior change problems are recognized (e.g., in public health, marketing etc.). Eliminating learning blockages is thus a crucial part of the behavior change task. The Behavior Centered Design (BCD) Behavior Challenge model (Figure 2.1) identifies a behavior change task for each step in the reinforcement learning process. These tasks are grouped, for BCD purposes, into three primary jobs that any behavior change intervention must achieve—Surprise, Revaluation, and Performance:

- *Surprise* is about the process of perceiving a stimulus via sensations and perceptions, with additional psychological responses, expressed as the problems of *getting exposure, grabbing attention,* and *facilitating processing.*
- *Revaluation* is about the parallel process of analyzing the stimulus for its value, via resources being acquired and valued in terms of rewards, which are the tasks of *modifying value* and *altering rewards* in behavior change terms.
- *Performance* is about the forward-chained process of establishing the best behavioral response to the stimulus via action selection and behavioral performance itself—by *getting selected* and *generating opportunities* for performance.

To reiterate, then, the challenge of behavior change consists of three basic problems (with two tasks for each):

- Create *Surprise.*
  - Get exposure.
  - Grab attention.
- Cause *Revaluation.*
  - Alter rewards.
  - Modify value.
- Enable *Performance.*

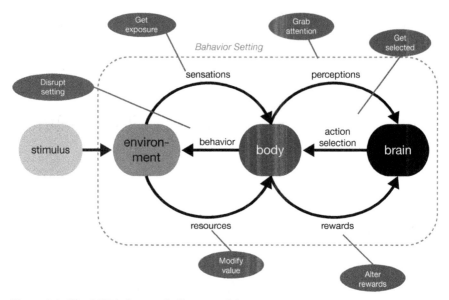

Figure 2.1. The BCD behavior challenge model.

- Disrupt setting.
- Action selection.

Solving these problems is a central focus of BCD. Each is discussed in some detail in this chapter.

SURPRISE

The first challenge in behavior change is to generate *surprise*. Most everyday behavior is settled into fixed patterns of response. To shake behavior out of these ruts, something new has to happen. So, if we are to persuade behavior into new directions, we first have to provide surprising stimuli. Let's discuss how surprise can be created.

Getting Exposure

If the immediate environment doesn't contain new stimuli, then no learning processes can take place and individuals will not respond to the intervention with changed behavior. Hence, the first job of any behavior change effort is to get new stimuli in front of people. Marketers tackle this problem by analyzing how and where their target population spends their time. They identify touchpoints— the places and times that they can exploit to connect people with products or to channels of communication [74]. For example, mothers with new babies may be targeted by pharmacies, while people looking at property websites may be targeted with furniture ads. A premium is charged for placing products besides tills in supermarkets or to use billboards on the side of heavily used transport routes. A touchpoint analysis in a rural low-income setting may reveal that clinics, despite being an obvious choice for health messaging, may be a poor channel of communication, as mothers may, on average, make very few visits each year to a clinic and then may only interact with a health worker for a few short minutes. Behavior change campaigns that do not get exposed to the target audience fail at the first hurdle.

Grabbing Attention

A second problem is that although people may be exposed to new stimuli, the stimulus may not be attended to, especially in message-inundated modern environments. Ensuring that the target stimulus gets processed is a design problem.

Luckily, we know what makes a stimulus stand out. We pay attention when we encounter a stimulus that confounds our predictive brain, when it seems that the world model in our heads may be wrong [75]. This means that we could be behaving inappropriately and possibly dangerously and that to fix the problem we need learn. So, a stimulus that we attend to is one that confounds what we already know and expect. For example, no one pays attention to small stones by a path, but when the same stone is moving in a trajectory likely to collide with our bodies, we respond immediately. No one pays much attention to a crowd of people queuing at a ticket barrier, but when one individual behaves unexpectedly, by doing a handstand, for example, we pay attention. Phenomena that defy evolved expectations are surprising. For example, phenomena that defy our mental models of how physical objects or biological creatures act, such as physical objects moving by themselves or nonhuman creatures talking. Think of seeing an ad containing a picture of a tree with eyes: trees are plants, but only animals have eyes, so a tree with eyes confounds expectations and, therefore, is surprising. In terms of the predictive brain hypothesis, this is called *prediction error*: we predict how we expect the world to be and pay attention when we find the prediction to be wrong, as it may mean that we have to fix something [75].

Producing a surprising stimulus is therefore what interventions should do, as such stimuli will grab attention. Creative people are good at coming up with surprising ideas, because they can think out of the box, which is why engaging creative people to help design behavior change programs is a good idea.

REVALUATION

Of course, a program's aims won't be achieved just by getting people to attend to a randomly surprising stimulus. Surprise must have consequences that result in desired changes to target behaviors.

So what sort of surprise will help us to achieve behavior change? We need to create the sort of new stimuli that will lead brains to think that the individual can get what they need by performing the target behavior. Brains are constantly scanning the environment for opportunities to employ behavior to get what the brain or body needs (or avoid what might harm it).

What are those things that we need? I will again turn to evolutionary theory to answer this question, because what we need, fundamentally, is to be able to survive and reproduce. So we have evolved to perceive value in doing things that present us with evolutionary benefits—that is, to engage in behaviors that produce resources that translate into improved chances of survival and reproduction. In essence, we are motivated (by expected value calculations) to pursue goals that will put us into these "good" situations. What is the nature of these good situations? The two basic evolutionary tasks can be further broken down into particular strategies, given the way in which humans live. For example, since we reproduce sexually, we must attract and bond with mates. Further, these bonds produce dependent offspring who must be nurtured. A full discussion of the different evolved human motives awaits in Chapter 3; for now, simply remember that there is a distinct set of motives that can be exploited in various ways by behavior change interventions.

Altering Rewards

So how can human motives be used to change behavior? One way is by emphasizing the rewards from performing the behavior or by highlighting the possible negative consequences. In both cases, the sensory salience, temporal proximity, or statistical likelihood of these rewards being experienced may not be obvious. For example, the spread of pathogens is imperceptible but nevertheless causes disease—a real threat that simply isn't easy to understand or identify using the human senses. By artificially making this process visible through exaggeration (e.g., the supersized bugs with evil personalities that appear in toothpaste ads inhabiting the mouth), the benefits of the behavioral practice can be made more salient.

Similarly, people may have the perception that rewards will only appear in the relatively distant future and, therefore, discount them in a way that is maladaptive. For example, the benefits of education may only be associated with getting a better job in the long-term future. But education can be revalued by emphasizing the good feelings associated with being more knowledgeable and capable in everyday matters now or by focusing on common expectations (i.e., simply doing what everyone expects of a young person).

Finally, the likelihood of experiencing desired rewards can be increased by offering guarantees of various kinds. For example, marketers often offer "money back if not satisfied" deals on new products to make reward statistically more likely.[1]

In summary, occurrence of a given behavior can be made more likely if the rewards that naturally follow from performing it can be altered by making the reward appear more or less obvious, more or less immediate, or more or less likely. However, this tactic may not actually change the amount of reward that is experienced from carrying out the behavior—only some perceived quality of it (e.g., how fast it is experienced or its sensorial richness). Hence, any revaluation may only be temporary. Actions may change once and then revert to the old pattern. However, we can do more than this; we can also change the value of the behavior itself.

Modifying Value

A key task for the would-be behavior changer is to modify the value of the target behavior. One way is via the classic marketing strategy of adding value to a product by adding a new association, for example, by suggesting the behavior is what high-status individuals (e.g., celebrities) do or by linking the behavior with a moral cause, such as suggesting that a brand is environmentally friendly or socially conscious.

All behaviors have a *proper domain* motive (i.e., that for which they evolved: eating assuages the Hunger motive, while the Hoard motive causes us to gather resources for a rainy day). However, other motivations can also be recruited to help instigate behavior change. For example, you can make eating an Affiliative activity or one that displays your Status. Indeed, through branding, values of all kinds can be added to a food: it can be portrayed as what good mothers feed their children (the Nurture motive) or as grown by local farmers (Affiliation motive). Obviously, the opposite can also be important: antismoking campaigns try to make smoking *less* valuable by suggesting that the practice isn't really popular among peers (i.e., not a norm in the Affiliation group) or only practiced by those of low Status, thereby *reducing* the number of motives associated with the behavior. By varying the number of motives and kinds of rewards attached to the performance of the target behavior, the new behavior is revalued and, hence, will become more/less likely.

PERFORMANCE

Despite getting attention, being processed, and engaging in Revaluation, the intervention must still get the target behavior to be enacted. The purpose of Performance is to interact with—and change—the environment in a way that minimizes Surprise as previously perceived—that is, to remove the perceptual error through behavior and thus make the look of the real world conform as closely as possible to the person's internal world model [75]. Performance of the target behavior should be the means by which this reconciliation between the individual's world model and the world itself is achieved. This problem can be split in two:

- Setting disruption.
- Action selection.

Disrupting Settings

Performance of the target behavior has to be perceived by members of the target population as a way to achieve the objective of minimizing the Surprise instigated by the intervention. This means that the context within which the target behavior occurs has to be modified in a way that causes the desired behavior to be part of the setting's mission. The basic rule is, Disrupt the context in some way so that the target behavior is performed. There are multiple ways in which this can be achieved.

While the Behavior Challenge model is precise about the psychological steps necessarily associated with behavior change, it is not specific about the nature of environmental influences (environment is left as a single variable). However, a very useful model of the environment is available in the form of the behavior setting concept [77]. A behavior setting is derived from the work of Roger Barker in ecological psychology [77]. Mealtimes, business meetings, air travel, educational classes, religious services, and waiting at a bus stop all constitute types of behavior settings. Such settings can be thought of by analogy to a stage play where actors congregate in a particular place to perform oft-repeated roles with certain props and well-rehearsed scripts. Each setting thus has a purpose, a designated place, a set of objects, and a prescribed set of behaviors. Each person entering into a setting expects the others who simultaneously participate in it to perform their (implicitly) designated roles. Deviation from these roles is generally punished by those participating in the setting.

To understand the power of settings, imagine that you are speaking in front of an important audience of your peers and you forget what you meant to say. In effect, you have failed to play your role properly, having been let down by your memory, due to the stressful situation. Those in the audience will express displeasure and annoyance, and you will attempt to recover as quickly as possible—your embarrassment being an internal censuring system to get you to perform properly. (For more examples of setting regulation, see the many videos of social disruption experiments on the Internet, which show what happens when people violate simple, everyday norms such as talking to or sitting too close to strangers in public place or not using silverware during a meal.) Settings are a powerful means of understanding what directs people's behavior. They suggest that we need to look to the supportive social conventions, physical objects, and infrastructure that regulate ordinary behavior. Behavior settings are the situations within which people have learned what to expect from the environment and from other people's behavior.

To continue with the theater analogy, a behavior setting can be said to have the following elements:

- *Stage:* the place and things surrounding where the setting regularly occurs.
- *Props*: the objects manipulated to help accomplish behaviors (often called *synomorphic* because they fit the behavior; e.g., a hammer is designed both to fit the hand and to bang in nails efficiently).
- *Infrastructure*: relatively large physical structures necessary for *performance* but that are neither manipulated nor damaged through use.
- *Roles*: the interacting strategies used by the cast of actors which meet their needs separately and together.
- *Motivation*: the motive(s) driving role-playing behavior in a setting (i.e., the goal or benefit an individual hopes to gain from playing a *role*).
- *Routine*: a learned sequence of behaviors performed regularly, and typically in the same order, to fulfill a role.
- *Script*: an individual's knowledge of a routine—that is, a set of mental instructions about how to behave (which may be implicit) in a particular behavior setting to play a role.
- *Norms*: the implicit rules governing role-play in a setting.

Changing settings is therefore a powerful and sustainable way of changing behavior [78]. Indeed, behavior change can be said to be essentially about *disrupting behavior settings so that appropriate learning can occur*. In effect, I argue that we must *reset* people's situations, so that they can naturally learn the appropriate thing to do.

Barker used cybernetic cycles to represent control mechanisms, operating not at the level of individual psychology, but at the level of the behavior setting itself [79]. His eco-behavioral operating circuits counter deviancies introduced by human or physical participants in the setting to maintain its progress through the setting's dynamic agenda. These are mechanisms for controlling the performance of settings, keeping people acting within their routines in conformity with their adopted roles, using objects in ways consistent with their synomorphic nature, and correcting deviations from the normal pursuit of the setting's objective. He argued that these control mechanisms reside not just in psychological processes, but also in the causal linkages between the physical, social and biological components of settings, making a setting a superordinate, dynamic, self-governing entity [80]. Thus, it can be argued that a setting is, essentially, a positive feedback system—like reinforcement learning itself—operating at a higher level of organization.[2]

One kind of setting disruption is role change—the strategic position played by some individual in a setting. If individuals pledge in public to adopt a new role, social control makes it harder for them to defect.

Attaching particular behaviors to the enacting of a role (e.g., via pledging) is one way to create new opportunities for the behavior to be performed. Pledging is making a commitment—preferably in public, to add weight to the promise—to perform the target behavior. It is also well-known that making the pledge specific as to the situation in which it should be performed—what psychologists call an implementation intention—makes it more likely to be performed [83, 84]. An implementation intention thus makes reference to particular behavior settings. Having people sign their pledge as well turns it into an implicit social contract, lending it further weight because failure to adhere to the contract can be punished by others.

Ensuring that the target behavior is performed may also require modification of the script for the setting. For example, people may currently think that getting their hands clean before eating simply requires rinsing them with water to remove any visible dirt. An intervention may suggest that this is insufficient because there are also dangerous but invisible agents that need removing from hands. To be effective, this intervention must ensure that individuals believe that the handwashing setting can only be successfully completed by including a new step in the routine: washing with soap as well as water. This means individuals must modify their script for this setting to include this extra step. Even if the step is omitted next time through habit, memory of the script may cause individuals to go back and insert the soap use before leaving the setting.

Another way of facilitating performance is to have people modify their environment by increasing the level of technological support for the target behavior. For example, installing an irrigation system makes watering the garden regularly much easier. Getting people to take their medicine is facilitated by buying a container with the time and day labeled on separate cells in the box, making it easy to determine whether this afternoon's dose has been taken or not. Simply putting the medicine out on the counter, rather than behind a cabinet door, can cause the medicine bottle itself to serve as a reminder. Such simple tricks can often suffice to increase the likelihood of performance when the setting arises. Similarly, the Target Setting can be modified such that some barrier to performance of an undesirable behavior is introduced, as when people stop having snacks in the house.

The target setting can thus be modified in many ways to safeguard that the target behavior is performed.

THE SETTING TRANSFER PROBLEM

There is a further problem, however: target individuals are typically exposed to an intervention in one setting (e.g., a community event) but perform the target behavior in another (e.g., sexual interactions in the case of an HIV program). For behavior change to occur, the individual must retain some mental novelty (e.g., an intention to perform the target behavior or a new associational value) during the period between exposure to the surprising stimulus and the time when opportunities to perform the target behavior occur. I call this the *Setting Transfer Problem*. It is another reason that behavior changers must ensure that the psychological effects of their intervention are long-lasting.

This problem is related to the issue in psychology called prospective memory, in which an individual must recall an intention to do something at a specific time and place in the future [85]. The prospective memory literature shows that the

Setting Transfer Problem can be overcome to some degree by making the intention to perform a behavior specific to a particular situation—that is, by couching the intention in the form of an implementation intention [86] or by placing reminders in the target setting that will help cue performance [87]. (Use of the word *performance* also purposely implies acting out or playing a role on a stage, which emphasizes that it occurs in a particular setting.)

The Setting Transfer problem can also be solved simply by creating some new mental association that is remembered long-term—that is, new information that comes to form part of long-term memory but that isn't a conscious intention. Just finding the target behavior more attractive because it is now linked (relatively permanently) to new, desirable goals (that satisfy other needs than the primary one) can work to cause the target behavior to be more highly valued.

This kind of processing—forming an intention or long-term memory—is more likely to happen if, at the time of exposure to the intervention, individuals

- have relatively few other stimuli to process (i.e., low cognitive load and low stress).
- have relatively more time before the next behavioral response must be produced.
- are in a social setting so that the experience can be shared.
- are in a teachable moment or life-change event (e.g., birth of child, moving), when they are seeking to learn how to behave differently.

These are all situational variables that can be modified by choice of touchpoint. For example, a doctor's waiting room may be a good touchpoint because people in the waiting room may be in a teachable moment and with time between activities. On the other hand, they could be stressed and, hence, unreceptive to new stimuli.

There are also ways in which the stimulus itself can be presented that make processing easier. These include employing

- multiple sensory channels to facilitate immersion (e.g., TV with sound and vision vs. radio, which is only sound).
- simplification and exaggeration of stimuli (as in animations) [88].
- highly recognizable settings to encourage rapid perceptual identification.
- narrative (i.e., using our evolved ability to process the simulated experience of others).

Action Selection

Even if all the previous steps have been taken, the target behavior may still not be enacted when an appropriate situation arises. This is because before a behavior is performed, it must be selected from among many other potential behaviors [62, 89]. That process can be delegated to the environment, as when a cue triggers an automatic habitual response. Alternatively, a motivated (although implicit) calculation may suggest that in the present state of hunger, consuming food has more value than hoarding it, for example. However, there are executive control factors that can also affect whether a behavior gets performed:

- *Cost*: the more expensive the action in terms of energy, time, and mental resources, the less likely it is to be performed.
- *Confirmation bias*: the tendency to value choices consistent with existing beliefs and values.
- *Availability* in memory of relevant information (e.g., one can more easily remember the name of a celebrity than a friend due to the former being heard in so many different contexts).
- *Endowment effects*: the tendency to devalue choices that require one to give up something that one has already acquired (e.g., to pay tax on income).
- *Locus of control bias*: the tendency to believe that exogenous environmental factors can be influenced through action.
- *Mere exposure effect*: the tendency to value things simply because they are familiar, not due to intrinsic qualities of the thing.
- *Fundamental attribution error*: the tendency to believe that others willfully choose to engage in behaviors rather than recognizing the power of the situation on them.

These biases and heuristics (or rules of thumb) for decision making have been investigated by behavioral economists, who see these as "predictably irrational" forces behind behavior [6]. Yet, from an evolutionary standpoint, all of these biases are rational, in the sense that they help people to make adaptive choices. For example, it makes sense to ascribe greater value to something one has possession of now than to a promise of the same thing later, since the future is always unpredictable and promises are not always kept. Similarly, the locus of control bias is often adaptive because it is better to assume that one is a forceful agent in the world than powerless, in which case no attempt at goal achievement would be made. For example, children with an internal bias (i.e., belief that events are due to their own, planned actions) function more positively and efficaciously in achievement situations than those with an external locus of control (i.e., those who believe events are primarily caused by factor external to themselves) [90]. The fundamental attribution error is simply the locus of control bias applied to other people, rather than oneself, and has a similar explanation: assuming others are responsible for their actions is a natural consequence of trying to predict others' behavior by imagining their mental states [91]. Further, overestimating the probability of others having aggressive intentions (and preparing a defensive response as a consequence) is a better error to make than assuming they are benign and risk exploitation or attack [92, 93]. The error can be explained as an appropriate bias when it reduces the costs of potentially dangerous inferences [94]. Thus, like behavioral economists, I believe these cognitive biases are operational in human decision-making, but unlike the economists, I argue that they are adaptive mechanisms. People should exhibit behavior that favors getting a reward now rather than later (i.e., temporal discounting) and make efforts to achieve goals in the face of obstacles (i.e., an internal locus of control bias) to be effective agents in the world.

The final valuation of a behavior is thus a function of the intrinsic value of the benefits received, as modified by the relevant action selection factors. The name of the game, then, is to make sure conditions are such that the target behavior wins in comparison to all other options after these factors are taken into account.

In Theory of Change terms, Performance can be considered the *outcome* of the intervention. As a consequence of having gone through this process of Surprise, Revaluation, and Performance, the desired outcomes should occur. These processes can be summarized in a central principle of BCD: *Disrupt settings with Surprise to force Revaluation and thus cause Performance.* This principle requires that the causal mechanisms linking the program implementation to the Target Setting in Theory of Change all work through as expected. In other words, the program design problem is to create an intervention that works like a guided missile, flying through the environment, ripping into bodies, and burying itself in brains, where it detonates, releasing repercussions that disseminate through the body and, via behavior into the environment, completing the learning cycle. As a result of the behavioral changes, the world should look more like the brain expects it to. If not, another round of behavior might be required to ensure that the world is a safe, well-known place, without any surprises in store.

This concludes my discussion of the basic theory behind the BCD approach to behavior change. However, the modeling thus far remains somewhat abstract in terms of the actual factors that might influence behaviors in the moment of performance. We still need to elucidate in greater detail what these factors might be, because it will be important when we actually come to the practice of identifying what aspect of the setting we need to change. Hence, we turn to the problem of behavior determination in the next chapter.

Behavior Determination

It is often useful to think about all of the things that can influence an individual's behavior at a given moment in time, rather than about the dynamics of learning (which has been the primary focus of the book thus far). For this purpose, the Behavior Centered Design (BCD) Behavior Determination model (see Figure 3.1) can be used.[1] It is essentially a representation of the reinforcement learning (RL) model from the previous chapter, but rotated 90 degrees, so that all of the components become overlaid visually on top of one another, capturing their causal relationships in a single instant, with the behavior setting remaining as a kind of "force field" linking the various components together. The brain is presented as being causally constrained by its presence inside the body, and the body, in its environment. Environmental and brain components have been divided into three categories to provide additional detail about the nature of these components. In particular, the environment is broken into social, biological, and physical components, while the brain is divided into executive, motived, and reactive (all of these distinctions will be discussed in the following text).

THE EXTENDED MODEL

As shown Figure 3.2, specific factors can be associated with each component of behavior determination, resulting in a checklist of factors to be considered in any proper description of behavior and examined by anyone attempting to intervene through a behavior change program.

A detailed discussion of the many elements of the Behavior Determination model is most efficiently presented as categories of factors that go into the BCD checklist. Each element has a precise definition, provided in Table 3.1, with examples. These categories directly correspond to the extended model (Figure 3.2). An example of a completed checklist is provided in the following text.

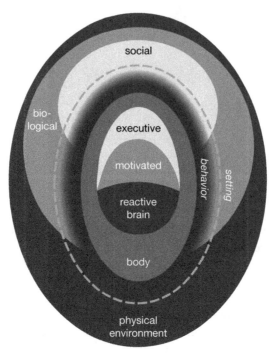

Figure 3.1. The BCD behavior determination model.
Source: Aunger, R. and V. Curtis, *The Evo-Eco approach to behaviour change*, in *Applied Evolutionary Anthropology*, D.W. Lawson and M. Gibson, Editors. 2014, Springer: London. pp. 271–295.

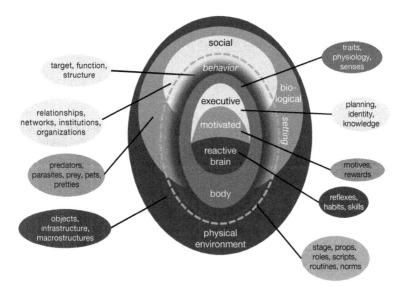

Figure 3.2. The BCD behavior determination model (extended).

Table 3.1. BCD BEHAVIORAL DETERMINANTS

Element	Definition	Examples
Behavior	A functional, dynamic interaction between the body and environment	
Target	Whether the behavior in question is the primary or secondary focus of the behavior change program	Primary, secondary, nontarget
Function	The type of evolutionary benefit provided by performance of the behavior	Reputation, food, knowledge
Structure	The hierarchical clustering of co-occurring behaviors	routines
Body		
Traits	Relatively permanent characteristics or behavioral predispositions	Openness, disgustability
Physiology	Aspects of body morphology (shape), size, and general body functioning	Gender, age, body mass index, metabolism
Senses	Specialized organs for acquiring information from the environment	taste, smell, hearing
Brain		
Executive		
Planning	Engaging in imagined evaluation of potential future events	Writing shopping list, daydreaming about being pop-star
Identity	A supra-setting narrative about one's place in the social world	Mother, writer
Knowledge	Consciously available, learned associations between specific concepts	Facts (George Washington was the first US President), beliefs (Unicorns look like horses except with a horn)
Motivated		
Motives	Psychological mechanisms to produce behavior that solves evolutionarily important tasks in the human niche	Lust, affiliation, status, create, hoard, hunger
Rewards	Benefits of unexpected value received as a consequence of behavior	Extra food or money, unexpected success in mating game
Reactive		
Reflexes	Innate automatic behavioral responses to environmental stimuli	Suckle, blink
Habits	Automatically triggered responses acquired through experience	Tooth-brushing, driving

(continued)

Table 3.1. CONTINUED

Element	Definition	Examples
Skills	A capacity to perform particular behaviors with facility developed through repeated practice	Hitting a ball, cooking a meal, giving a speech
Environment	The causally exogenous factors impinging on behavior	
Social		
Relationships	Dyads with special psychological significance to participants	friend, neighbor, colleague (at work)
Networks	Personal, but informal clusters of people	bridge partners, "tennis club members that I meet socially"
Institutions	Sets of behavior settings linked by a common purpose, often occurring in a common place	Market, marriage, club
Organizations	Formal institutions, with rules/ regulations/policies for converting roles into positions and for excluding/ admitting individuals into specific roles	Business, club, guild
Biological		
Prey	Species that are consumed by people	Food species (plant and animal)
Predators	Species that consume people	Lions, bears
Parasites	Species that crucially depend on people for survival and reproduction	Pathogenic bacteria
Pets	Species that humans have domesticated for companionship, not consumption	Dogs, cats
Pretty things	Species that humans have domesticated for aesthetic pleasure	Flowering garden plants
Physical		
Objects	Relatively small-scale, rapidly improvable physical implements which are often significantly affected by use (and hence are prone to obsolescence or destruction)	Ball, soap, watch
Macro- structures	Large-scale systems that have an indirect causal impact on behavior (e.g., delivering the water that is used to wash hands with soap); tend to be super-setting-sized, but to intrude into settings in particular ways	Systems: water supply, electricity grid, road or computer network; mega-structures: skyscraper, dam
Behavior Setting		
Stage	The place and things surrounding where the setting regularly occurs	Bus stop, a restaurant

Table 3.1. CONTINUED

Element	Definition	Examples
Infrastructure	Local structures that directly facilitate or constrain behavioral performance while not being affected through use; typically circumjacent to the behavior setting (i.e., encapsulated within the setting stage); mid-sized structures that are not manipulable (at least by a single individual) but that nevertheless play an important role in a setting	Table, room of a building
Props	The objects used to accomplish behaviors within a setting	Dinner-plate, fork, knife
Roles	The interacting strategies used by the cast of actors that meet their needs separately and together	Waiter, chef, customer
Routine	A learned sequence of behaviors performed regularly, and typically in the same order, to fulfill a role	Enter restaurant through front door, walk to table, sit down, study menu, interact with waiter, etc.
Script	An individual's knowledge of a routine; that is, a set of mental instructions about how to behave (which may be implicit) in a particular behavior setting to play a role	Choose a table, order Food, eat, pay at the Cash register
Norms	Implicit rules governing role play in a setting	Don't leave restaurant without paying

BEHAVIOR

Behavior is an evolved adaptation. Plants can't do much in the way of physical movement beyond following the sun around with their leaves.[2] Animals, when they evolved, developed purposeful and dynamic interaction with the environment to get what they need [96]. This is what I call *behavior*. Animals that produced the behaviors that were best able to extract resources from the environment or avoid its dangers produced more copies of their genes in subsequent generations. These genes also reproduced the brains that generated these adaptive behaviors in their offspring. The behaviors themselves wrought adaptive changes to environmental conditions. Indeed, the purpose of behaving is to extract benefits from the environment or to avoid dangers that might lurk there. One might even say that animals co-evolve with their environments via behavior [14, 97].

Behaviors need not be produced independently, one after the other. Rather increasing levels of control over the production of behavior leads to multiple actions being produced together to achieve more hard-to-reach end-states. The result, from an observational point of view, is that these actions become statistically and functionally correlated (i.e., chunked together) in time and space [98–100]. Much of behavior therefore has depth, or structure, in time because a number of behaviors can be clumped together by our brains and produced as a group in sequence, thanks to motivational- and executive-level control (see following discussion; also see Box 3.1).

Choosing the right behavior in a given circumstance is thus a major computational problem. Luckily, another adaptation evolved to solve that problem: hierarchical RL (see Box 3.1).

Box 3.1.

BCD THEORY

Behavior Sequencing and Reinforcement Learning
Behavior occurs in an ongoing stream, as people move through their environment or produce streams of audible output. Behavior streams can be organized hierarchically into very long units (getting an education), long units (going to school), short units called episodes (finding coat, saying goodbye, and getting bicycle) and very short, unconsciously executed units (taking a step) [101]. These different scales of behavioral chunking coincide with the routine, scene, event, and action hierarchies found in the literature on routine behavior [102]. We have also adapted to parse our observation of these movements into events and higher-order chunks [102, 103] or, in the case of speech, to perceive the stream of sounds as words and sentences [104],[7] Further, this chunking of behavior into higher-order units can occur recursively, so that a multilevel hierarchicalization can be performed, leading to quite complex behavior patterns being controlled with relative efficiency in the form of daily routines.

The RL model has been augmented to deal with hierarchically organized behavior. This is because standard RL models are subject to the curse of dimensionality. According to the basic model, an animal can only learn to behave adaptively by engaging in trial-and-error learning. As a result, the time needed to arrive at a stable choice for action selection increases with both the number of different end-states in the environment and the number of available actions required to achieve those end-states. In fact, the total number of actions needed to explore this space can increase exponentially. In a human context, with a complex environment and many behavioral options available, this would suggest that the standard reinforcement learning model quickly becomes computationally infeasible [33].

One way to combat this scaling problem is to introduce hierarchical control architectures [105, 106]. In hierarchical RL, sequences of actions can be grouped into subroutines, each of which is evaluated according to its own subgoals. Thus, rather than select among a set of elemental actions, interpreted as relatively simple motor behaviors (such as grasping a spoon, scooping up some sugar, and depositing the sugar into a cup), hierarchical RL allows the agent or animal to perform multiaction routines containing sequences of lower-level actions, casting them as a single higher-level action or skill (such as "add sugar") [37]. These sequences, called options, have their own subgoals. If a subgoal is not met, it generates its own prediction error. These pseudo-reward prediction errors may not be associated with actual resources, but with achievement of an internally generated subgoal that is but a stepping stone toward the desired outcome. Nevertheless, the agent is motivated to reach these subgoals, once the option gains control over behavior. Attaining the subgoal yields a special reward signal, referred to as pseudo-reward, which serves to sculpt the options policy. Placed within a hierarchical framework, pseudo-reward prediction errors are used to learn which combinations of actions reliably lead to a subgoal, while reward prediction errors are used to learn which combinations of subroutines lead to rewarding outcomes [107]. It appears this is how learning in the human brain occurs as well [108, 109]. In particular, prediction error responses at different levels of a hierarchical learning problem appear to recruit the same dopamine-based mechanisms—that is, dopaminergic responses seem to control learning from internal subgoals as well as from end-goal achievement [110]. RL with temporal differences can thus be applied to domains with both sequential and hierarchical structure. Significant effort has therefore gone into the development of RL algorithms which are specifically designed to operate in this kind of hierarchical context [105, 111, 112].

Because they are associated only with the small number of actions in the subroutine, pseudo-reward prediction errors substantially reduce the complexity of learning. By introducing intermediate subgoals and arranging these into recursively more abstract structures, hierarchical RL can explain the kinds of complex behaviors humans produce.

In fact, this discussion suggests the dimensionality problem of RL is not really a problem once evolutionary and ecological reasoning is adopted. In particular, our investigation into the environment shows that it can be highly refined in practice, because a niche only has a reasonably small number of dimensions, reducing the number of factors to which an animal must actually pay attention. Only a few biological species fall into relationships with humans (e.g., millions of insect species go unnoticed by humans), while imitation is a common way of reducing the dimensionality problem in the social environment: simply copy what others are doing [29]. I have shown that the physical environment is also concentrated into a few infrastructural complexes and focal objects to support specific behavioral performances. Further, behavior itself is often controlled as hierarchical routines, which leads to a major reduction in the number of end-states that must be considered, while behavioral settings constrain the ways in which these different components can interact in particular circumstances, so that only a few kinds of actions are likely. Thus evolutionary and ecological constraints significantly limit the conceptual space that trial-and-error based RL must explore to reach adaptive action selection outcomes. In real life, people make use of multiple kludges that turn RL into a tractable option for guiding even complex behaviors.

BRAIN

Evolutionary processes designed the brain to produce the adaptive behavior that makes use of opportunities and avoids threats in the environment [25, 113, 114]. More formally, the brain seeks to be in a low energy state, in which all its expectations are constantly being met by circumstances [15]. However, when something new and unexpected is encountered in the environment (e.g., because a behavior setting has been disrupted), this implies that the brain may no longer be producing the optimal behavior, so attention must be paid to seizing the new opportunity or to avoiding the new threat. If the new situation is dealt with effectively (i.e., the behavior it produces in response results in a positive goal state), a reward signal in the brain causes that new behavior to be reinforced and, hence, repeated when the opportunity presents itself again. This constitutes an episode of RL by the brain. Eventually behavior settles down into a new pattern, when what the brain expects is no different from what the environment offers. A new habit may even be formed as the new behavior becomes a part of the normal routine. The brain has had a learning experience (i.e., changed its model of how the world works in some way), and it settles down into a new low-energy state where everything is again predictable.

The human brain is composed of 100 billion neurons, each linked by around 7,000 synapses to other neurons, forming a network of incredible complexity; it is one of the most complex objects in the known universe. Nevertheless, there is a growing consensus that how the brain works can best be described using a simple proposition: it makes predictions about the world it lives in and acts to correct mistaken expectations about how the world works [115–117]. The human brain can thus be called a prediction-generating (and error-correction) machine [15, 33, 52, 118]. It has been designed by evolution to produce realistic expectations about what might happen as a consequence of engaging with its environment via behavior. From this perspective, the job of any brain is to minimize the size and number of prediction errors it makes about the consequences of its own actions. This requires the brain to have a good idea of how the environment will respond to its own behavior. That is, it must understand the environment to predict what the environment will do. Note that although the human brain is often called the most complex thing in the universe, this is a very simple way of describing what it regularly does with a single optimization algorithm: the brain is about minimizing its own prediction errors by developing the best possible behavioral policy.

The brain doesn't just passively react to situations (so, the standard psychological word of *response* is something of a misnomer) but rather carefully monitors its situation and engages proactively whenever something unexpected is perceived. It is thus constantly making predictions about what the external conditions should be and, whenever there is a discrepancy, seeks to correct it via behavioral interaction with the environment.

Three Levels of Control

The predictive brain deduces what is the best strategy in response to disruptions of behavior settings, but the production of adaptive behavioral responses is controlled in three different ways: via reactive, motivated, and executive mechanisms [96]. (See Box 3.2 for an explanation of how the different mechanisms of control over behavior evolved in humans and the following section for an explanation of why these distinctions are classes of RL.)

REACTIVE BEHAVIOR

First, behavior can be purely reactive—a rapid, automatic response to a stimulus, without conscious awareness. In evolutionary terms, this is the first type of behavior to have arisen and has been present since animals first evolved. Examples include a flinch response to feeling a burning match or a learned automatism such as changing gear while driving up a hill. Reactions learned through repeated experience are called habits [162], and much of everyday behavior is produced in this way [133].

MOTIVATED BEHAVIOR

The second type of behavior to evolve, in invertebrates, was motivated behavior. Motivated behavior is directed toward the achievement of evolutionarily beneficial goals. This direction is provided internally to the brain and body by the reward system, which provides indicators of progress toward, and achievement of, goal-states. Reward signals in the brain tell us that we are on the right track and teach us to repeat rewarding behavior but not to repeat behavior that produces the opposite: signals of punishment. Specific mental mechanisms have evolved to produce this goal-directed behavior, which we call *motives*.

How do motives shape our behavior? An animal, driven by hunger (one of the 15 evolved motives characterizing animal behavior), may seek to savor a novel substance, but unless the taste experience is rewarding, the behavior of eating that food will not enter the animal's repertoire. Such rewards guide animals on the way to beneficial end states (in this case, having consumed appropriate nutrients). Rewards can include sensory pleasures (hedonic sensations such as taste or smell) as well as metabolic benefits for the body (e.g., rising blood glucose levels from food consumption).

Rewards both guide behavior along the path to meeting needs and also kick in when the end-state is achieved (i.e., when a need is met). Rewards may or may not be consciously felt. So, for example, although saccharine and sugar may both feel sweet and rewarding to the tongue, the lack of physiological impact on blood glucose of the saccharine may make it less rewarding overall and, hence, less likely to be employed habitually than sugar [163].

The human way of life involves solving specific kinds of evolutionary problems, which were set by our niche, such as finding food or a long-term mate or ensuring we are treated fairly in social dealings. Motives are evolved psychological

Box 3.2.

BCD THEORY

The Evolution of Behavioral Control

The brain is an evolved organ adapted to produce behavior that promotes survival and reproduction of its body [25, 96, 113, 114, 119, 120]. As such, it has a long evolutionary history during which it has acquired a variety of adaptations. Primary among these are mechanisms for controlling behavior. Three levels of control have evolved in human brains, each of which can be isolated neuroscientifically [121–125]. The points at which these different control mechanisms evolved are crucial steps in the development of behavior production in humans. Responses to behavior also take the form of learning and memory mechanisms associated with each level of control.

The baseline for behavioral control came when early invertebrates such as jellyfish and worms appeared (about 600 million years ago). The first control mechanism to have evolved, and which remains characteristic of invertebrates, was simple reactions to environmental stimuli that likely represented opportunities or threats. This is Pavlovian decision-making, which entails the release of species-specific approach and avoidance reactions in response to unconditioned or conditioned stimuli (i.e., reflexes) [126]. So, recognition of a potential food item would inspire approach among these early animal species and contact with a poison would inspire recoil [127, 128].

Among these relatively simple nervous systems, learning is restricted to basic forms of conditioning, or acquiring associations between stimuli or between stimuli and behavioral responses [129, 130]. The result is incremental learning of relatively inflexible stimulus–action relationships that are released upon exposure to certain environmental stimuli. This reactive-level learning is based on the Hebbian rule whereby neurons that "fire together, wire together" [113], such that associations become stronger through experience. For example, in fear conditioning, an animal acquires avoidance responses to a previously neutral stimulus when it becomes paired with an aversive stimulus, such as a shock or loud noise. Reactive level learning is called "classical conditioning" by animal behavior researchers. It involves attaching a new link to an existing cluster of knowledge (e.g., feces tastes awful, so the animal will recognize feces next time as something to avoid tasting). It is Pavlovian in the sense that the learning is to associate an unconditioned stimulus (bad taste) with a conditioned one (the sight of feces). Such learning is also predictive in the sense that feces will now be expected to taste bad whenever it comes into view, even without the experience—a learned aversion [124]. A special form of Pavlovian learning is evolutionary-prepared learning mechanisms such as the Garcia effect, a mechanism that trains the body to avoid poisonous substances after only a single exposure, due to its significance for survival [131]. These acquired (rather than innate) automatisms are commonly called "habits" [132, 133].

The first novelty in behavior production occurred with the arrival of mammals around 200 million years ago. The psychological adaptation characteristic of mammals is motivational control for goal achievement [134–137]. Goals are mentally represented end-states that the brain calculates can be achieved through some sequence of behaviors. The existence of goals enabled new forms of learning because satisfying the goal can be accompanied by psychological rewards that promote the same behavior the next time the situation arises. This is achieved by associating the positive outcome with whatever mental mechanisms produced the behavior in the first place (i.e., evaluative learning). For example, signals from peripheral parts of the body can be sent to the brain to indicate the current status of various tissues and organs (e.g., hunger) that instigate searches for an improved state (e.g., food consumption). In this way, animals can learn a potentially arbitrary behavioral policy to obtain rewards or avoid punishments (e.g., a rat can learn to press a lever in one location so that food becomes available in another location). Learning can now rely on mental representations, or clusters of associations, so that associations between clusters constitutes a higher-order form of associative learning. Goal-states can come to be associated with the characteristics of events that lead to occurrence of the desired end-state; these characteristics make the goal more or less salient (e.g., waterholes may become associated with capture of prey if prey are often successfully encountered at waterholes) [138, 139]. This style of learning will be called *affective*, as it is designed to help animals achieve rewards via goal satisfaction. It uses the temporal difference error rule discovered by RL researchers to associate the animal's current state with its degree of progress toward the current goal, working sometimes with respect to mentally represented states that only have psychological value, not resource value (i.e., a state that is leading the animal to, or correlated with, achievements of a state that will provide resources).

Emotional memory is associated with affective learning. It is a facility for storing affectively charged experiences and associations, particularly those representing significant opportunities or threats and, hence, likely to produce large rewards or punishments [140–142].

Also associated with the development of a reward system and goal representation are motives, or psychological adaptations for achieving particular kinds of goals. These goals are associated with solving elementary evolutionary tasks such as finding food or a mate. Which motives a species can be expected to exhibit are determined by the niche in which the species lives, which, in turn, define the evolutionary problems it must solve to flourish and reproduce [96]. All animals must find food, many must find a mate (if they depend on sexual reproduction), and fewer must climb the social ladder of status (because only a few animals are social, much less have social hierarchies). The means by which each of these niche-based tasks is solved depend on the species' evolutionary history (e.g., some species solve the food problem by scavenging; others, by being predators). The various human motives will be described next, as their roles become relevant.

When primates evolved about 65 million years ago, a third level of control arose, called executive control, based on the ability to run through imagined scenarios of future outcomes. This deliberative level of decision-making entails search and evaluation of action options through a representation of the causal structure of the world [143]. This can be thought of as occurring through recursive test-operation–test-exit units operating on hierarchical mental modules [144], a straight-forward application of the cybernetic principle on which RL is built.

In RL terms, executive level learning is instantiated as an actor-critic model (a member of the class of model-based learning mechanisms) [32]. The actor is the map (or database of world knowledge), which gets feedback from the reward system, so it learns new facts about the world (e.g., where food can be found or more declarative memory items), while the critic (equivalent to the temporal difference-based system, which executive level mechanisms makes use of) updates the expected value of the just-performed behavior, based on the same reward feedback signal as is fed to the actor. Thus, the executive level just adds the actor part to the motivational system. Executive level learning is more about new memory resources than new learning mechanisms.

Learning at this level can be associated with hierarchical goals, or subgoals that represent achievement of mid-states that reflect some conceptual or functional clustering (e.g., being the first stage of a process that results in resource acquisition, such as boiling a pot of water for tea). Goals at any level of the hierarchy are evaluated using the same temporal difference error mechanism as works at the motivational level.

Some of the processing occurring at this level bubbles into consciousness, which is a limited theater in which memories and other information are pulled together for decision-making and other tasks [145]. Declarative memory is a specialized mechanism for remembering the specifics of particular experiences, such as the license plate number of the car that just hit someone on the street or the name of a second cousin [146, 147]. Declarative memory allows humans to develop highly specific scenarios based on detailed information and thus weigh up very complex chains of potential future actions against one another. Identity is a special form of declarative memory—a stored representation of the self (a cluster of associations about the person and its history). For behavior change, another important form of memory is social norms: people have ideas (based on experience) about what other people do (descriptive norms) and what other people think they should do (prescriptive norms), which can impact on their own behavior (through the motives to affiliate or increase status).

Thus, for each level of mental control over behavior, there is an affiliated adaptation for the storage and recall of information specific to the control task at that level. There is also a specific mechanism for learning at each level, which at the executive level is conceptual learning. This is a recursive form of earlier learning, in that it now can work with even more deeply embedded mental representations, such as a model of the self placed within a model of the external world. Learning can also come from the conscious rehearsal of recent failures or successes or from the rehearsal of possible future action sequences, using our strong narrative-producing mechanisms—something called *reflective learning* [145, 148].

All three behavior-determination or control systems are operating all the time, in parallel, to not waste experience. Having multiple decision-making systems allows the brain to make use of controllers with different advantages. Model-based learning (forward search) is a good policy when close to reward (i.e., there are few steps to be searched) and there is little time for training; model-free learning (relying on cached knowledge) is more appropriate when the individual has lots of experience and the distance to reward is not too important. Reactive-level behavior determination is best when there is little margin for error (e.g., the consequences of a wrong decision impact on morbidity or mortality). So, a general rule is, if an animal has experienced only few trials of a particular circumstance, it should use executive level production (because it will be able to produce some estimate of the likely returns to behavior by searching the relevant solution space); if it has more experience, it should use learned automatic responses (i.e., habits). On the other hand, if prior generations have had similar experiences, their correct responses might have been encoded in Pavlovian reactive mechanisms producing hard-wired responses [149].

Thus, with each increasing degree of sophistication over the production of behavior, there are psychological adaptations for selecting among more and more complex sequences of behaviors, which can be put together based on information recalled from specific forms of memory that store just the kinds of information needed to construct those mental representations of future activity. But this means there is competition at any given moment between them. Thus, there must be some mechanism for integrating between them (i.e., a meta-control mechanism). There is growing evidence that they are integrated [122, 150]. The control of behavior can be shifted from one system to another through focal brain lesions, suggesting the coexistence of neurally distinct decision-making systems [151, 152]. Choice between systems is to trust the one that is more confident of its recommendation (i.e., habit when lots of experience and low uncertainty, model-based when opposite conditions), so getting expected value with uncertainty [47].

All of these evolutionary developments through the phylogenetic history of our species can be seen as outcomes of the RL algorithm in action over thousands of generations, producing a wide variety of adaptations in nervous systems and the environment, as well as interactions between these phenomena. Note that all of the early adaptations persist in our species and should continue to characterize human behavioral performances.

There are also significant interactions between levels of control over behavior production and evaluation. In particular, habit formation is a specialized mechanism that progresses control through each of the three levels of control through repeated experience [153–155]. It can begin with a conscious decision to acquire a new behavior, progress to motivated behavior, and, through continued learning in regular environments, end up as a practiced automatism. Over time, repeated temporal-difference learning can lead to reduced errors, at least in stable environments, until the errors are essentially eliminated, at which point the brain releases control to reactive level production (i.e., the response becomes habitual) [156]. This is Thorndike's law of effect [157]. In each step, repeated reinforcement leads to reducing the level of control necessary for continued behavior production, ending up with fast-acting, automatic responses to environmental cues using a purely reactive mechanism [158]. With this kind of Pavlovian control, actions are automatically elicited at the presentation of reinforcers, whether the actions lead to acquiring rewards or avoiding punishments [124, 159]. In humans, procedural memory is an adaptation to help recall the skills necessary to execute what have become automatic behavioral responses [160, 161].

Other interactions between control mechanisms like this no doubt await discovery. However, these complexities can also lead to problems. Reactive, affective, and reflective learning mechanisms can interact in complex ways that introduce structural constraints on learning. Interactions among these various brain structures can constrain learning in ways that lead to maladaptive outcomes, regardless of changes in the environment, as they have evolved to serve different ends and then been forced to work together. Alternatively, some forms of interaction between complex RL mechanisms and environmental stimuli, or unexpected endogenous responses by the environment to behavior, may also cause problems. Thus, kinds of difficulties that lead to a need for behavior change can arise within the brain, in the environment as a stimulus for learning, or in environmental responses. Interactions of various kinds among the elements of the BCD model (or even within a structured brain) can thus be the source of a need to change behavior.

---

mechanisms that help us to choose the appropriate behavioral response to a situation—that is, the response most likely to lead to a satisfactory outcome, as measured in evolutionary terms (of gene survival and reproduction) [96, 164, 165]. For example, we are motivated to

- avoid bad smells because they may betray a disease threat (Disgust).
- give a present to our lover because it may help keep them around to help rear children (pair-bond love).
- take free offers even for things we don't need (Hoard).
- work to advance our social standing (Status).
- avoid threats of predation and accidents (Fear).

Each of these motives helped our ancestors survive and compete in our evolutionary past.

Motivated behaviors often come at some short-term cost, in terms of physiological effort, time, or just missed opportunities to achieve other, easier goals. For example, an animal might undergo immediate discomfort (like climbing a tree) to seek out a rare source of food such as honey. Or they might invest in play behavior if it equips them with social or manual skills to rear children or fight their conspecifics. (For a more complete description of the human motives see Box 3.3; a full history and description of each motive can be found in a recent book I co-authored with Val Curtis [96]. (Note that the word for each motive has a technical meaning derived from its evolutionary purposes, which does not always correspond exactly to the lay terms used to name them.)

Box 3.3.

BCD THEORY

Human Motives

Motives can be derived from deductions about what kinds of goals are important to a species, given the way it lives. The set of human motives therefore reflects the particular set of evolutionarily important tasks humans must perform to survive and reproduce. Drives are those motives that provide direct changes to the state of the body; emotions are motives that modify the state of the environment in ways that facilitate later satisfaction of drives, and interests are motives whose primary function is to provide information to the brain that can be used to eventually satisfy needs. The following figure sets out the full suite of human motives, showing at what stage each one evolved in our ancestral lineage.

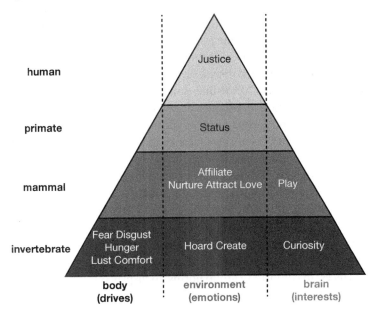

Drives

   Comfort. Because terrestrial niches vary in terms of physical conditions such as temperature, elevation, and moisture levels, maintenance of the body's physiology requires behavior such as relocating to shade when the sun is hot; covering the body with warm, dry clothes and finding shelter when it is cold; removing thorns; tending injuries; and saving energy by sleeping.

Hunger. Like all organisms, humans have basic metabolic needs to sustain bodily tissues. These are met through the acquisition of resources such as nutrients, water, oxygen, and sunlight.

Fear. Humans, like most animals, face threats from the environment. Fear drives behavior that avoids "hurt from without" threats, including predators, but also aggressive conspecifics and the chance of accidents like falling from a cliff.

Disgust. Animals also need to avoid "hurt from within" threats (i.e., parasites), which are able to sneak undetected into the body. This motive causes the avoidance of bodily fluids, sick others, off foods, disease vectors, and contamination. It has been linked to our reasons for avoiding people who violate social norms as well in the form of moral disgust.

Lust. The need to maximize the production of gene copies in the next generation causes people to engage in copulatory behavior, because humans reproduce through sexual intercourse. This requires a search for and pursuit of appropriate candidates and the consummation of sexual union.

Emotions

Nurture. Mammalian offspring are born dependent, requiring provisioning, protection, and education. Nurture is the motive to rear offspring and aid kin. The Nurture motive drives feeding, cleaning, and protective behavior; providing opportunities for play learning; and attempting to influence the social world in favor of kin (nepotism).

Attract. Humans have to compete for mating opportunities. Making sure one is attractive can help secure one-time copulations or long-term pair-bonds. It causes individuals to produce displays of sexual attractiveness through body adornment, painting, or modification; provocative clothing; or through activities that display mate quality such as sport and dancing.

Love. Human mothers need to keep men around long enough so that they can share the burden of rearing highly dependent offspring. Love causes both males and females to invest in a pair-bond that ensures this investment with tactics that include making costly gifts, offering tokens of commitment and the jealous driving away of rivals.

Affiliate. To gain the benefits of group life, humans invest in membership in groups. We are motivated to participate in social activities, to form alliances, to conform to group norms, to display our intentions to cooperate, to seek to engender trust, and to share resources, including knowledge about others.

Status. In hierarchically organized groups, individuals seek to enhance their relative social position so as to have priority access to resources. This is achieved by tactics such as flattering superiors; submitting to authority;

drawing attention to one's one contributions; displaying wealth, ability and cultural taste; and seeking recognition and title.

Create. One's habitat can be improved such that it is more conducive to survival and reproduction. Tactics include building dwellings that are safe and dry; removing dangers such as predator or parasite habitat; planting, weeding, and irrigating; cleaning, tidying, and repairing habitat; and making artifacts such as bows and ploughs that aid the diversion of energy toward survival and reproduction.

Hoard. Actions can be taken now to ensure that resources are available later, when they may be required, but less readily available. Hoard motivates behavior that involves the accumulation of resources, either directly by growing, collecting, and storing or, more indirectly, by negotiating the rights to territory or the fruits of group production. It may also require the guarding of resources from pilfering by others.

Justice. Only humans live in very large groups of unrelated individuals. Cohesion in such groups appears to be regulated by people's willingness to punish not only those who mistreat them, but those who mistreat others in the social group. The Justice motive causes humans to enjoy punishing those who behave antisocially.

Interests

Curiosity. Because the environment is constantly changing, it is necessary to update one's information about current conditions. The function of the Curiosity motive is to collect and codify information, thus reducing a gap in knowledge about some facet of the world. Curiosity motivates exploratory behaviour and results in brain structures being created or updated, such as world maps and situational expectancies.

Play. Time can sometimes be spent acquiring skills to be used later in contexts important to biological fitness. Play drives the acquisition of embodied skills and knowledge of one's own physical competencies through the repeated practice of particular behaviour sequences. Play-driven behaviors involve simulating activities such as nurturing babies, fighting, hunting, or courting, without its related dangers.

PLANNING AND EXECUTIVE CONTROL

Finally, higher primates have a third means of producing behavior. They can use executive control to plan beyond the time horizon of immediate reactivity and short- to medium-term motives. They can imagine alternative futures, evaluate which are likely to be most beneficial (still valued in terms of reward), and hence plan to do something even more beneficial. For example, they can sacrifice the opportunity of an extra-pair mating by imagining the consequences for their family or forgo the opportunity to attend a party for the sake of getting better marks on an exam, both of which may have greater payoffs in the long term. Humans (and possibly some other animals) can even direct their own thinking processes consciously to make decisions about what to do next—the highest form of behavioral control. Most efforts at behavior change have focused on addressing this rational deliberative brain, on the assumption that it is primarily in control. However, new evidence suggests that this part of the brain is reserved only for particular types of situations [166, 167]. Most behavioral decision-making is, in fact, carried out elsewhere, in automatic conformity to scripts and routines in behavior settings and in the comparative valuation of routes to goal states, weighed in the currency of reward.

SUMMARY

What are the implications of the three-level brain for changing behavior? First, habits, by their nature, are hard to institute, but if habits can be created, they are likely to persist. Second, motives can be harnessed to drive the behavior in question. If disgust of dirt and contamination is an important driver of hygiene behavior, then perhaps it can be harnessed to increase handwashing, as has been done successfully in several interventions I've been associated with [168, 169]. If a behavior occurs publicly, then perhaps it can be made a token of Affiliation— what "our group" does—and, hence, rewarding. Third, while we like to think that the top-level brain—the one that carries our conscious rational planning—is in charge of our behavior, mostly it is not. Long-term plans are weak in the face of immediate temptation and often give way to habits. The best way to use our rational brains to change our behavior may be to find clever ways to trick our habits and motives—by placing cake out of sight or not buying it at all when one wants to diet, for example.

RL Models and Levels of Control

It is worth noting that the predictive brain viewpoint provides explicit foundations for my basic claims about mental operations. In particular, there are three families of RL models from studies in neuroscience and animal behavior that conform to the three types of behavioral control identified by BCD.

First, the policy-search family of RL models is equivalent to our Reactive level of control. This type of model involves the immediate use of a response policy: depending on the assessment of the situation, it just chooses a response from a predefined suite of possible responses (the so-called policy set)—equivalent to inborn reflexes—or chooses an action based on some average value function, previously learned that represents the aggregated experience from many previous trials (which is the equivalent of a habit). Neither of these responses explicitly represents the actual outcomes or contingencies in the task: they simply are preferred actions or summaries of some prior valuation that react to the agent's current situation (and a history of experience in that situation). As a consequence, like stimulus-response habits, they cannot be adjusted if the appropriate end-state happens to change, because there is no representation of a goal [122, 170, 171].

Second, value-function-based RL models correspond to the motivated brain; these models engage in a search for actions that maximize value, using the temporal-difference algorithm to evaluate progress toward a goal. Value-function models attempt to find a response that maximizes the agent's return from behavior by maintaining a set of estimates of expected returns from all the available options. This kind of model does evaluation based on the agent's current position or situation, but looks only at possible options from the current position, evaluating each in turn (it doesn't look backward) [111, 171]. Given its cached estimates of the value to be returned from each behavior, it chooses the one with the highest value.

Finally, model-based RL is the way the brain's executive function operates: it encodes how likely each possible outcome is and can learn an internal model of probable consequences of being in some state. That is, it learns state transition probabilities [33, 172]. This kind of model can do both forward and backward tree-like searches through all possible outcomes to find the best strategy. This can be considered to be more about learning than immediate use, as it can also optimize over the longer term aggregate rewards rather than single-goal achievement. The model can infer the likely value of alternative future courses of action based on any situation (not just its own current one), which is the primary function of imagination. Sophisticated model-based algorithms explicitly compute a separate transition matrix for the probability of ending up in each next state, given the current state and each possible action choice [33, 173]. This resembles human planning, which can be used to find an optimal generated (rather than pre-existing) policy over several sequential goals, and hierarchical model-based RL speeds up this learning process by chunking potential behaviors into event sequences.

These different types of control are presumed to all be available in the human brain, operating in parallel. The system that produces the least uncertainty about what the highest-value option is wins the competition to instruct the body what the next behavior should be (i.e., their action gets selected in the action-selection sweepstakes) [122, 174].

BODY

Brains wander the world inside bodies. Their job is to take good care of the body they are in, making sure the bodies survive and reproduce themselves. But brains can't do this directly; they have to make bodies do the job themselves in the end, by collecting resources from the environment.

Bodies have evolved adaptations to ensure they can extract resources in optimal fashion. Humans in particular have specialized abilities for extracting resources. For example, the body's opposable thumbs (among other features) help to create the complex machines that can extract more resources than muscle-power itself [175–177].

The body is our primary interface with the environment, how we modify our surroundings, through behavior, to better suit our needs. Two aspects of the body are important when considering how it produces behavior. First, any body has a morphological nature; that is, its precise shape and structure determines what sorts of movements that can be undertaken. For example, the body's size in part determines how much force can be applied to environmental objects (e.g., how far a stone of a certain weight can be thrown). The precise shape of the beak of the various Darwin's finches determines which feeding niche they occupy, as it determines which sorts of nuts and seeds can be successfully consumed [178]. Internal body morphology is also relevant. Thus, reptiles and birds produce eggs, which need specific forms of care and defense as compared to the live offspring produced by mammals. For these reasons, there tends to be a tight relationship between body morphology and a species' niche.

Once we get to humans, however, each body morphology, being unique and visible to others in the social group, also gives people an ethnic, gendered, age-grouped identity, which is stored and modified by experience in declarative memory (the kind of memory associated with executive control). Social roles are important as part of identity as well and became individuated with the multifarious division of labor that accompanies membership in the large groups that humans live in. This identity can also include psychological aspects: cultural beliefs, traits of various kinds (such as personality and mood), and episodic memories from one's personal past (a specific form of declarative memory). These are obviously psychological in nature but arise as a consequence of the body's unique appearance and experience. Similarly, long-term biases in the performance of behavior (e.g., mood, personality-based traits) can also be thought of as being associated with the constancy of the body, rather than the constant turmoil of the brain, and so as having some physiological element (e.g., as reflecting general excitability) [179, 180]. Skills, or the ability to perform highly practiced behaviors well, such as athletic feats or complex everyday behaviors, are also often thought of as embodied, given that they become embedded as muscle memory in the peripheral nervous system [181].

The body produces physiological changes in response to signals from the brain that action is imminent. Arousal can be considered as part of the metabolic system from this perspective. Arousal is increasing activation of the autonomic nervous and endocrine systems, leading to increased heart rate and blood pressure and sensory awareness in the presence of a threat or opportunity in preparation for action. It is also a way the body prepares for goal pursuit [182–184], so it can be considered an adaptation arising with mammals to energize motivated action. Arousal is the body's endogenous response to information from the brain about an action having been selected.

Second, engaging in movements such as behavior requires physical energy, which, in turn, requires mobilization of the body's chemical machinery for producing kinetic energy—that is, the body's metabolism. The body thus experiences an energy drain as a consequence of engaging in behavior; against this, it can acquire resources (e.g., through prey capture).

Causation is also reversed in the sense that the brain is impacted by residing in a body. For example, RL can reflect embodiment, taking place specifically with reference to which parts of the body help achieve goals; that is, the algorithm can be modularized to include multiple reinforcement processes for each relevant part. For example, when actions are produced via simultaneous movement of both hands, a model suggesting left and right hands received separate reward feedback for each hand movement produced better predictions of chosen behavior than a traditional model that treated the actions as unitary, with a single value [185].

Remember that behavior is defined as the interaction of a body with its environment, so the body is the brain's instrument for effecting change, and this colors the way the brain works in fundamental ways. Many researchers now admit that the brain's activity is heavily influenced by its presence within a body. The field of embodied cognition has grown up around this insight and demonstrated many ways in which this dependence plays out [186, 187]. For example, when people are asked to think about things that might happen in the future while sitting down, they tend to lean forward slightly, while if asked about past events, they tend to lean backward [188]. This kind of bias extends to perception itself, as the very first responsibility of the brain—to detect opportunities and threats—depends on the ways in which the body can provide information about the situation via various senses. For example, desirable and threatening objects, both of which require behavioral responses, appear closer than comparison objects, which are not likely to be interacted with, a phenomenon called "motivated distance perception" [189]. The embodied cognition point of view is consistent with the predictive brain perspective as well [190]. Essentially, the relationship can be framed as the brain modeling itself as an agent embodied in an environment, harvesting sensory evidence in support of that model of its external world and forming hypotheses about how to effect changes in it.

Although most behavior change theories ignore them, bodies can be important in behavior change. For example, when the target behavior is obesity, changes in body morphology can be an indicator of program success; when it is an anti-smoking campaign, physiological dependence on certain chemicals can be a significant factor to take into consideration when designing the program.

BEHAVIOR SETTINGS

Bodies interact with their immediate environment through behavior. Behavior is a dynamic interaction in time and space. This means that it is a situated phenomenon. However, situations are poorly theorized, with little agreement as to how they should be categorized or even which dimensions are relevant for such a classification [191–193].

This would be a calamitous state if there wasn't actually a more powerful concept available to fill this gap: the portmanteau concept of a behavior setting (see Box 3.4) [79]. In humans, behavior almost always takes place in repeated, predictable contexts, with recognizable features. These situations can be described as behavior settings [77]. As suggested earlier, disrupting these settings is key to

Box 3.4.

BCD THEORY

Behavior Settings

A behavior setting is a recurring situation composed of people interacting with their environment to fulfill an emergent function in a particular time and place [77]. This emergent function is associated with the typically social nature of settings. Performance in a setting can be thought of as execution of a "we plan"— that is, an implicitly agreed social contract among members of a temporary social network to perform coordinated behaviors together, thus achieving goals that it would be more difficult for individuals to achieve on their own [194]. Behavior settings can be considered the (still-evolving) products of cultural evolutionary processes for establishing the best ways of getting everyday jobs done. Indeed, they are probably a human elaboration of the rites and rituals in other animal species associated with evolutionarily important tasks like attracting males and competing with other males or for territory. Elaboration comes in the fact that the behavior sequences associated with settings can be much longer and less rigorously defined (i.e., more flexible). Repeated performance of a role within a recurring setting gives people the chance to find the most rewarding and efficient means of fulfilling the needs that can be satisfied by that role (which then becomes their personal script for how to perform in that setting).

Behavior settings are thus networks of constraints on how animals behave in specific situations. The first manifestations of settings appear in the form of rituals and routines.[8] The everyday activities of many animals are characterized by the stereotypical repetition of specific behaviors in particular sequences. It is well-known that major life events such as mating or territorial disputes proceed in a ritualized fashion—that is, using conventional signals and accentuated body movements— to secure the best outcome [196, 197]. These are situations of high risk and high reward in evolutionary terms; hence, appropriate behavioral responses have been strongly selected, so that the best outcome can be most reliably secured. These adaptive responses are again likely to be the same, given a stable environment, so that they can become quite rigidly produced, perhaps by specific rules of response. Most animals, from ants to lizards to primates, also have daily routines in which they choose the same places and times to conduct a particular behavior (e.g., feeding, getting water, marking territorial boundaries, resting, sheltering), day after day [26, 198, 199]. Since RL results in optimal behavioral choices over time, then as long as conditions remain essentially the same, the same options should be chosen, and the same behaviors observed—hence, the high degree of stereotypy in many animal behaviors. Behavioral rigidity, such as the preference to engage in specific acts at particular places and to take familiar routes between these places, is adaptive because it allows faster performance and requires less attention, enabling attention to be directed to other potentially varying aspects of the environment, such as the presence of predators [200–203].

Humans have elaborated such settings to a significant degree, thanks to the ability to play particular roles, often facilitated by modified physical infrastructures. A given behavior setting often involves people interacting with focal objects (e.g., a Bible), specific kinds of infrastructure (e.g., a church building), and people playing complementary roles (e.g., choristers, parishioners, lay leaders). People can (often simultaneously) enter into an implicit contract to complete the execution of a particular setting, such as a church service, school class, shopping trip, sporting event, or private routine. Each participant plays a particular role within the setting, helping the group to achieve the setting's purpose, which may be to entertain (e.g., a Broadway show), educate (e.g., a biology class), acquire resources (e.g., a business strategy meeting), or avoid some danger (e.g., a fire drill). Playing a role typically involves performance of a particular sequence of behavior to facilitate completion of the behavior setting's function or task (e.g., the leader of a religious service leads the other participants through a sequence of events with symbolic significance). This can be considered one of the setting's *routines*.

Each role involving taking a particular position within the setting that is more or less central to the function of a setting. For example, a church service would be difficult to complete without a pastor to conduct it, and the organ player is also quite important but not as central as the pastor, while having a person to greet parishioners at the door is a functional luxury in many cases. It is often not necessary to refer to psychological states to predict the sequence of behavior someone playing a particular role in a given setting will exhibit, so powerful are the regulatory pressures that dictate proceedings within settings [204].

Because these processes interact through bodily development, brain-based learning, and environmental modification, there can be consequences that are the result of this coevolution itself. That is, aspects of the environment can be adapted to the way brains and bodies work. Objects and infrastructure involved in settings often have design features that facilitate or invite the performance of certain kinds of behavior—that is, they can be a component of asynomorphy [77, 205].[9] This is a specific relationship between a person and an object, facilitated by the object's design, in which use of the object facilitates performance of a particular behavior. For example, chairs help people to rest while remaining vertically oriented for work or social interaction. Synomorphies are adaptive kinds of fit between environment, brain, and body. For example, a bar of soap has a number of features that enable it to remove dirt from hands. It is about the size of a hand so it can be readily picked up and rubbed; it is relatively solid, so that it will last a long time yet, when wet, bits can be removed through easy friction to be left on the hand, at which point further friction will cause the bits of soap to foam, providing easier transport of dirt from the hand when washed off under a flow of water. All of these represent aspects of a synomorphy between the bar of soap and the human hand.

Our view of behavior settings is also explicit about the conceptual linkages between Roger Barker's work and that of Irving Goffman on social occasions [206] and the latter's dramaturgical interpretation of face-to-face social interactions [207]. I therefore use terms like *stage, script,* and *role* rather than Barker's original (and rather more idiosyncratic) terminology. Goffman was aware of the conceptual link from settings to game theory as well, in which the *moves* of an individual are dependent on those of others in the *game* [208]—an important formalism for understanding the strategic interdependencies operating during behavior setting performance, as those performing their roles properly depend on others doing the same simultaneously (e.g., when engaged in cooperative activity like eating at a restaurant).

---

behavior change. For example, in a food hygiene intervention in Nepal, groups of neighbors came together for kitchen makeovers, in which the kitchen space was repainted and decorated as a safe food zone, food preparation gadgets were distributed, and new behavioral scripts were agreed to between them—all of which succeeded in creating new, safer food preparation routines among mothers in the intervention villages [78]. Adding value to unrewarding target behaviors by incorporating them into treasured social roles reinforced their performance.

Settings involve dynamic, adaptive interactions between most of the components of the BCD approach already described. As a result, settings are physically ephemeral in nature, like behavior itself. Understanding how these components work together requires sophisticated investigations of the control mechanisms that manifest themselves through the dynamic interaction of brains, bodies, and environments. For example, anyone who begins to engage in behaviors outside the remit of their role in a setting, such as causing a disruption in a classroom, will be punished (e.g., by being told to leave the room) so that the other participants can achieve their goals. Such regulatory mechanisms can be discovered by observing them in action [79]. In social settings, this means that people performing their roles can help to train others to perform theirs more appropriately—in effect, socially reinforced behavior change.

ENVIRONMENT

Behavior always takes place in some environmental context. But there are aspects of the environment that are important to the performance of the target behavior in its setting, and others that are not. For example, having a coffee in a coffee shop depends on coffee cups as props, the water supply as infrastructure, the coffee shop employees and customers playing their complementary roles, etc. On the other hand, the achievement of the behavior setting's mission is not defined by, nor directly dependent on, how much oxygen is in the room, whether there are a few microbes on the tables, or the color of the paint on the walls. These relatively extraneous aspects of the environment are considered as conceptually belonging here, rather than as part of the behavior setting per se.

In parallel, it is, of course, important to explore what can be thought of as macro-environmental or contextual factors. What other programs and activities are occurring (or have occurred) in the target area that might compete with or be complementary to the planned program and thus assist, or interfere with, the Theory of Change mechanisms? Could a handwashing program be piggy-backed on an existing vaccination program, for example [209]? Could the marketing of one product be coupled with that of another to achieve economies of scale for the company? These contextual factors, including the general political, economic and social climate within which the program has to work, can influence program outcomes, and so should be taken into account during formulation of the Theory of Change as well.

Unfortunately, the notion of environment remains indistinct. In ecology, habitat, biome, and ecosystem are all quite vague concepts, largely defined by the geographical features and ecological community in the area predominantly inhabited by a species (e.g., montane, aquatic, alpine). In evolution, the idea of a niche—taken as a set of dimensions important to survival and reproduction—remains more abstract than is useful in the context of changing behavior. At best, the niche has been conceptualized as a hypervolume or multidimensional space of resources such as nutrients, territory, or mates used by organisms to satisfy fundamental biological needs [210]. What we require is a way of gaining focus on levers and triggers of change that are extrinsic to people, or outside.

One way of moving toward a more precise definition of *external factors* is to divide environmental phenomena into three types—physical, biological, and social—as a function of how they influence behavior. This division is supported by the sort of response that these different types of environment make to behavior. First, the physical environment responds in simple Newtonian terms to behavior: if you kick a stone, it flies away until its momentum dissipates.[3] An animal, on the other hand, can be strategic in its response, such as when a rabbit avoids being caught by a predator by scampering in random fashion across the landscape. Finally, a component of the social environment, another human being, will respond in potentially very elaborate ways to a simple stimulus—for example, forming a life-long plan to get revenge for a perceived wrong (e.g., the Count of Monte Cristo). Because these responses occur in different ways, human brains should perceive and respond to physical, biological, and social factors in the environment differently when producing behavior. Indeed, it appears that different kinds of deductions are commonly made with respect to physical, biological, and social objects, as suggested by the literature on folk physics, biology, and sociology [211–214]. For example, physical and biological objects can be distinguished in three ways: physical objects are not expected to have internal motivation, while biological objects are [215]; biological objects are embedded in unique hierarchies (i.e., the tree of life), while artifacts can be in several hierarchies at once [216]; and animals don't have specific purposes (e.g., tigers are not "for" anything in particular), but artifacts do (e.g., hammers are for hitting things) [217]. So these three types of environment are real in psychological terms and, hence, should be distinguished in behavioral models.

Two other types of argument also support this tripartite division: evolutionary and ecological. That is, the physical, biological, and social environment also differ in genetic terms: the physical environment doesn't contain any genes, the bio-logical environment (other animal and plant species) have a different gene pool from us, and the social environment is the current manifestation of our same-species gene pool. A final perspective is ecological, which makes reference to a species' niche. Conspecifics have the same niche (roughly speaking) as the focal individual, while members of other species will have at least somewhat different niche to live in. However, physical objects aren't restricted to a specific niche at all but can exist anywhere on the planet's surface.[4]

Physical Environment

We can use evolutionary principles to draw further distinctions and to trace the development of these three different types of environment. Two aspects of the physical environment can be distinguished in technological terms relevant to behavior [218]. First, in most cases, as we previously discussed regarding the top public health problems, the behaviors public health workers are interested in changing typically involve manipulating a technological object to facilitate the behavior's performance—for example, condoms for safe sex, soap for proper handwashing, and seat belts and air bags to avoid casualties in car accidents. Similarly, in marketing, the behavior change problem is to increase use of par-ticular products, which also tend to be objects, such as shampoo, telephones, and automobiles. In all cases, these are relatively small-scale, rapidly improvable phys-ical implements that are often significantly affected by use (and, hence, are prone to obsolescence). Objects are thus aspects of the physical environment that are manipulable and tend to decay or get damaged as a consequence of use (e.g., chair, soap, hammer, laptop) [218]. Focal objects are thus key to the performance of many of the behaviors people seek to change. Invertebrates have been shown to manipulate objects [219, 220], so this connection between behavior and objects has had a long evolution.[5]

A second aspect of the physical environment is also specifically adapted to producing behavior. However, it evolved to a very modest degree in other primates and significantly only in humans: what I will call *infrastructure* is the consequence of long-term niche construction, conducted by human beings, often over generations.[6] Infrastructure is the "big stuff," often called the *built environment*—things like a city's electricity grid, roads, skyscrapers, or the World Wide Web. It consists of modified aspects of the environment that are relatively inert or stable when used, remaining in roughly the same state, leading, in part, to their durability [218].

Thus, infrastructure and objects respond differently in endogenous terms to behavioral interaction. Recognizing the dimensions of functionality in an object or infrastructure can help when thinking about how the technology it-self can be modified to increase its ability to perform this function or how its use can be modified by the person handling it to make use easier or more rewarding.

Biological Environment

Our basic model of the biological environment is fairly simple, as any animal only adopts a few behavioral relationships with other species (see Table 3.2). In particular, there are three ecological relationships: an animal can be predator or prey to other large-scale animal and plant species or serve as a host or vector to pathogens, which eat from the inside. Each of these relationships is associated with a specific psychological motive: Disgust helps us to avoid becoming a host (or vector) to parasites; Hunger is designed to maximize our intake when we are acting as predators on plant and animal species; and Fear (via the fight–flight–freeze mechanism) evolved for dealing with the proximity of predators (i.e., to help us avoid becoming prey). All of these relationships involve a biological agent passing through the body boundary in some form (e.g., by being eaten, taking a bite of the person, or infecting the individual as host). More generally, Curiosity leads people to explore their physical surroundings to ensure they have up-to-date information on all available threats and opportunities, which are primarily about locations of food, potential predators, and pathogen habitats.

More recently, however, humans have developed *cultural* relationships with other species. First, some species are used as products or to provide services (e.g., trees are grown for wood; corn, for fuel; sheep are used for wool; a donkey, to pull a cart). These are species we treat as if they are physical objects. Second, some species we see as pretty and wish to have within view for aesthetic reasons, such as flowering plants and swards of grass, perhaps because they remind us of our ancestral condition in the African savannah [222]. These are species we treat as if they were part of the physical infrastructure. Third, other animals serve as pets: animals we keep in close contact without eating, because we are fond of them. These are species that are treated as if they were members of our own species. Thus, each

Table 3.2. TYPES OF RELATIONS TO OTHER SPECIES

Name	Relationship	Motive	Examples
Ecological			
Predators	Eats you from outside.	Fear	Bear, lion
Parasites	Eats you from inside.	Disgust	Bacteria, viruses, insects
Prey	You eat it.	Hunger	Cow, cereals
Cultural			
Products	You use it.	[Treat like physical object]	Biofuels, transport animals, trees as wind-break
Pretties things	You tend it.	[Treat like physical infrastructure]	Flowering plants, grass
Pets	You keep it for companionship.	[Treat like social object]	Dogs, cats

kind of cultural relationship to other species constitutes a perversion of a different kind of relationship to the environment, either physical or social.

Social Environment

The human social environment has become more complex than the biological one. Most invertebrates don't have a social life, being born and then abandoned to their fate almost immediately. Mammals were the first large-bodied animal group to spend a significant proportion of their lifespans in the presence of conspecifics, with whom they had particular kinds of relationships. However, mammals didn't develop significant structure within their social groups, which remain largely egalitarian in nature. Primates were the first in our evolutionary lineage to develop hierarchical societies, in which there is privileged access to resources, including mates [223, 224].

Humans have developed social life to a unique degree. We live in very large groups that can be composed of multiple subgroups. Some of these typically meet in particular locations, with associated infrastructure, such as businesses, governments, sports clubs, and religious organizations. Such organizations or institutions can be considered forms of social technology that facilitate new kinds of cooperative outcomes. Each of these can be thought of as a network of individuals linked through particular kinds of relationships, in which each individual is playing a particular kind of role, to help that organization achieve its designed ends. These networks can have regular kinds of structures (e.g., an organizational chart with a pyramidal shape) that dictate the ways in which it is possible to change roles within the organization (e.g., through appointment to a higher-status job by consensual agreement among others in the group).

More generally, social groups form *networks*, or structures within which one takes a place or position (e.g., social roles). Within these networks, there can be specific *relationships*, which are enduring dyadic interactions (e.g., mother–offspring). Playing a given role in an organization, network, or relationship can involve activation of a particular motive. For example, Status maximization drives some people to become CEOs of businesses, while pleasure in skill development (the Play motive) leads others to become professional sportsmen. Play has also been extended in primates from object play to social play for learning the skills to interact with conspecifics effectively [225]. Affiliation is the motive to simply belong to a particular group, to share membership with others in a common goal [165]. Brains, bodies, and adaptive behavioral responses thus evolved in tight lockstep with environments.

CONCLUSION

This completes my discussion of the set of factors that the BCD approach suggests can account for the determination of human behavior. Those seeking to change behavior would do well to consider the entire suite of factors as potential constraints *and* facilitators of the behavior targeted for change. This is obviously a lengthy list, but human behavior is incredibly complex and multifaceted, which is why targeted behavior change can be difficult to achieve, especially at the scale of populations. However, I believe that use of theory, as developed here, can reduce the difficulty and uncertainty associated with identifying appropriate means for achieving change, which brings us to the question of how to practically accomplish this goal—a challenge dealt with in the second part of this book.

PART 2

Practice

I now come to the problem of translating this theory into a means by which behavior can actually be changed, typically by a group of interested parties with a particular goal in mind for some target population or organization. However, at minimum, the situation could be someone looking to change their own behavior (as in self-help efforts). I will use a public health program development process as my central example in the following chapters, but similar steps and processes apply to any behavior change context (as I discuss in the final chapter through a number of example scenarios). A more detailed, step-by-step guide to the program development process is provided in the BCD Manual, found on the Behavior Centered Design website (https://www.lshtm.ac.uk/bcd).

The Program
Development Process

How can an individual ensure that their motivation to change will result in new, stable patterns of behavior in their daily life? How can a company get the biggest sales from a new marketing campaign? How can a public health program use resources most effectively to shift the largest number of people in a given population into the healthiest behaviors? Behavior change problems come in many sizes and shapes. Nevertheless, I argue that all of them can be addressed by following a similar process: designing new stimuli that get around the learning failure associated with undesirable outcomes.

However, programs that aspire to change behavior need to do more than just understand the active ingredients that will enable appropriate learning and, hence, performance of target behaviors. They also need a methodology for designing, delivering, and evaluating behavior change programs. We therefore now move to a focus on how behavior settings can be purposefully disrupted to achieve some desired change in behavior. The diagram in Figure 4.1 will be used to introduce the approach. This is the Behavior Centered Design (BCD) process model. Across the middle of the diagram is the chain of events that has to occur for any behavior to change. In a nutshell, an intervention has to change something in the environment, which has to change something in the brain and/or body of the target individual, which then has to influence behavior. The aggregate of these individual behaviors then has an impact on some state of the world (i.e., the factor the project aim seeks to affect, such as some population-level health indicator or global sales of a product). This causal chain represents the BCD approach to defining what is known as a Theory of Change. (For more background on Theories of Change, see Box 4.1.) This Theory of Change model, shown in the following diagram, is another way of representing the reinforcement learning model discussed in Part I as the intellectual foundation of BCD.[1]

The middle of Figure 4.1 highlights three key tenets of BCD (described in Chapter 2)—*Surprise*, *Revaluation*, and *Performance*, concepts that figure importantly throughout this book—and what links these together are the behavior setting in which they occur.

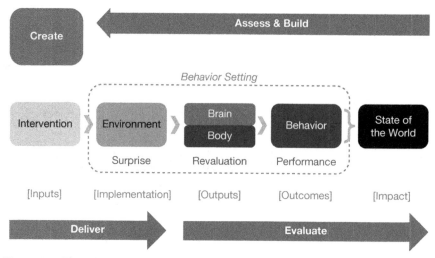

Figure 4.1. The BCD process model.

The five steps of the BCD program development process are depicted along the top and bottom of Figure 4.1. I have dubbed these the ABCDE steps, as follows:

A: *Assess.* Here program designers start by gathering what is known about the target behaviors, the target audience, the context, and the parameters of the intervention. A framing process leads to a statement of what is known already about how change can be achieved and sets out hypotheses about change mechanisms for further exploration.

B: *Build.* Build involves carrying out carefully targeted formative research with a sample of the target audience to find out the things that are unknown and explore hypotheses about the likely drivers of change. Unlike typical formative research, which involves key informant interviews and focus groups, BCD employs a variety of innovative methods such as motivational mapping, product attribute ranking, scripting, and video ethnography in a rapid deep dive with target audiences. The insights from this formative research are then ordered into a Theory of Change and distilled into a brief for the next phase.

C: *Create.* The Create step involves a creative team iteratively designing the intervention package and testing it on a small scale. Creativity is hard to package into a simple process, but it is vital if interventions are to be engaging and motivating enough to stand out in the crowded lives of those targeted by programs. The result of the creative process is a package of surprising and disrupting intervention materials designed to have maximum effect on the target behavior.

D: *Deliver.* The intervention package is then implemented via a set of planned activities, which may involve direct and indirect contact via

Box 4.1

BCD Theory

Theory of Change

Theory of Change is an emerging approach to guiding program development, execution, and analysis [226]. It is a term of art used in program evaluation circles that is similar to the older concept of a logic model or logical framework (logframe) but that is more focused on causal claims. Having an explicit Theory of Change helps one to think clearly about the pathways by which change occurs, to design interventions that are more likely to affect those pathways, and to better evaluate how program inputs have led to the desired outcomes and impacts [226]. It requires that program managers make explicit assumptions about the cause–effect relationships between program activities and behavior change, about the operational/logistical expectations for delivery of those activities, and about the macro-environmental context within which the program is taking place. This allows program stakeholders to attribute results to program activities when both the program and the context are complex (a useful ability in the era of evidence-based policy) [227]. A Theory of Change can be used in several ways: as a process description that makes explicit the causal connections between program inputs and outputs, as a strategic planning tool to guide action, and as a conceptual or thinking tool from which to learn from experience [228]. BCD uses a particular version of a Theory of Change that is focused on behavior. As Figure 4.1 shows, three causal links must be made: from Surprise to Revaluation to Performance (which result in changes to the state-of-the-world that the program seeks to influence). Since Surprise, Revaluation, and Performance are glosses on implementation, outputs, and outcomes, the BCD model demonstrates a tight connection between a fundamental learning process and a clear Theory of Change—an integration not previously achieved in the Theory of Change literature. Having a Theory of Change also helps with delivery and evaluation, so that lessons can be learned and extrapolated to other contexts.

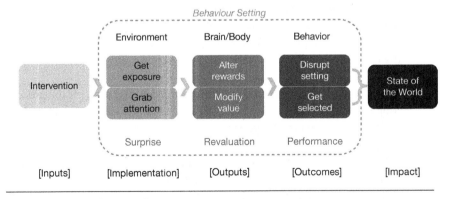

various channels such as community workers, events, and mass and/or digital media that are appropriate to the audience and intended impact. This process is monitored to ensure that learning from this experience takes place.

E: *Evaluate*. Ideally, the Evaluate step takes place in a field trial at a scale that allows some definitive assessment of whether the processes expected by the program's Theory of Change have taken place. The learnings from evaluation should then provide the starting point for a new cycle of learning by engaging in the BCD process again to develop a new program.

The BCD process model (Figure 4.1) displays the development process steps A, B, and C along the top, and the execution steps D and E along the bottom. Development is conceptually a backwards mapping process with respect to the Theory of Change: beginning with a long-term aim (i.e., impact) and working backwards through a chain of mechanisms toward the earliest changes that need to occur, the introduction of an intervention. In backward mapping, one builds the outcomes pathway starting at the most general and longest-term outcome and then drills down by identifying each set of preconditions, ending at the most particular, immediate, and short-term outcomes to be achieved.

The process I set out here is not unlike many others used in the development of, for example, personnel training (e.g., the US Army ADDIE [analysis, design, development, implement, and evaluate] model [229]), humanitarian responses (e.g., the United Nations' Coordination of Humanitarian Affairs model [230]), organizational capacity-building (e.g., the United Nations Development Programme model [231]), software, [232] or public health programs (e.g., the PRECEDE–PROCEED model [233]). Each of these models tends to have somewhat different sets of steps (e.g., the United Nations Development Programme capacity development model consists of engage, assess, plan, implement, evaluate), which makes it difficult to know how to choose the most effective process from among the many similar candidates. I argue that the BCD process consists of the minimum set of necessary and sufficient steps for designing and conducting an effective program. Each step is necessary because program executions that ignore or skip a step are less likely to achieve an impact. And the steps are sufficient, because they progress from the beginning of program definition to the end of program execution and analysis.

As with any project, it is essential to form a core team that oversees the process. Marketing experience suggests restricting this team to a stable set of six to eight stakeholders and behavior change experts who anchor activities and seek specialist support when needed.

Here I set out an ideal version of the overall BCD process. What I describe could employ considerable resources, many experts, and a long time frame (e.g., a year) and would be warranted for large investments. However, smaller programs should also follow each step in some form, as it is the logic of this process that produces results in terms of behavior change at the end. For example, a project may not be able to conduct formative research, but this doesn't mean that the functions normally performed during the Build step shouldn't take place—in particular, there still should be some design process in place.

My description is also ideal in the sense that while I have partitioned the process into a number of steps that are sequence-dependent to some degree, there can be conceptual and temporal overlaps between them. For example, baseline data collection might occur prior to the beginning of intervention delivery (i.e., while some elements of the intervention are still being Created). The steps should be seen as functional/conceptual in nature and not as completely isolated, with clear beginnings, middles, and ends. Many aspects are iterative. For example, the research design for the Evaluate step needs to be thought about from the very beginning and revisited during each step in the overall process. It can even be tweaked after implementation by revising the strategy used to analyses implementation data.

I have also indicated explicit outputs for each step in the form of reports of various kinds (e.g., Formative Research Protocol, Creative Brief, Process Evaluation Report). However, explicit reports about the framing process (in the Assess step) or implementation (of the Deliver step), for example, are often not written in actual practice. Nevertheless, I have used this device to indicate what sort of conceptualizations should have taken place in relatively final form at a given point in the BCD process. Thus, at the end of the Create step, program managers should have a clear idea about how the intervention will be delivered, to whom, by what means, with what intensity, and using which component materials. I gloss this as an Implementation Plan. The materials themselves (e.g., posters, TV ads, event guides) should also be ready for use. This does not mean that such plans have not been contemplated before this point; that Implementation Plans cannot be tweaked, even during the Deliver step; or that materials can't be modified in the face of evidence that they are not having the desired effects. In this respect, my description is also a simplification, as I often don't explicitly discuss how iterative modifications of concepts, plans, or materials occur; I only note that in real-world cases such complications often happen. My rule here has been to assign

---

Box 4.2

BCD Example

Introduction to the SuperAmma Program
Throughout my discussion of the BCD process steps, I will illustrate principles with an example. The SuperAmma Campaign was a project funded by the Wellcome Trust with the objective to use a theory-based handwashing behavior-change program to reduce child mortality due to diarrheal disease in rural India. (SuperAmma is "SuperMom" in Hindi; see www.SuperAmma.org.) Look for subsequent example boxes to follow this story along.

---

landmarks to the points at which a given process should be mature. Box 4.2 provides an example.

With this overview of the program development process, I now move on in subsequent chapters to describing in more detail how each step of the BCD process is used to develop behavior change programs.

Assess

The Assess step sets out the scope of the program and identifies what is known about the target behavior(s). First, existing information is collated concerning the determinants of behavior, and, second, this information is developed and organized into a Theory of Change via a framing process. This provides the basis for the next step, Build, which addresses any remaining gaps in knowledge required by the developing Theory of Change.

BACKGROUND REVIEW

The Assess team first determines what is known already by conducting, or commissioning, a background review that collates existing knowledge related to target behavior production. It may be possible to locate previous formative research in the country, or from elsewhere, to provide good insights into the drivers of current behavior. For example, in the SuperAmma project (introduced in Chapter 4), we reviewed the findings of formative research into handwashing behavior in 11 countries and were able to draw out many insights. For example, we learned that disgust and the perception of local handwashing norms were important factors in driving handwashing around the world [234]. In a nutrition project in Indonesia, we learned from reading previous formative research of a culture of frugality, with families keen not to "waste" money on food [235]. Key informants present at a framing process for another project in Zambia were able to explain that although most mothers knew that they should breastfeed exclusively, very few did so, helping us to rule out lack of knowledge as a reason behind poor rates of exclusive breastfeeding [236]. Hopefully, from the background review, program managers can determine which sort of learning failure underlies lack of performance of the target behaviors and begin to think about the basic strategy for overcoming this barrier.

FRAMING PROCESS

Second, stakeholders and experts work together to frame the overall task and agree as to what is known and what is still be found out, typically in a short framing meeting or workshop.

To ground program development in practical reality, it is useful to create a straw man intervention—a rough, preliminary idea of what the behavior change program might look like, taking into account known constraints (time, capacity, resources). The Behavior Centered Design (BCD) process model diagram is used to draft an initial Theory of Change: what are the desired impacts, behavioral outcomes, changes in brains, environments, and settings and how might this causal cascade be brought about through an intervention?

Filling in the Theory of Change (the central part of Figure 4.1) requires answering a number of questions:

- *What* is the aim of the program? (i.e., the *state of the world* the program wants to improve)? What precisely are the current and the target behaviors?
- *Who* is in the target population?
- *Why* is the behavior performed (i.e., what psychological mechanisms cause it to be enacted)?
- *How* can the target individual's situation be influenced so that they might be induced to change their behavior?

I next describe the answers to each of these questions in more detail—in reverse order, based on the Theory of Change, because that is the way the causal links are built up.

State of the World

Determining the ultimate aim of a program is typically the starting point of program design. It typically reflects the fact that a problem has been recognized that is in need of change. The aim often lies beyond behavior itself and typically concerns bringing about change in some state of the world (in the most general sense). Different kinds of states of the world can be relevant here:

- The power or ability to achieve an objective (e.g., easier access to health facilities, strengthened organizational responsiveness, increased social capital, increased government funding, improved self-control in the face of temptation).
- The state of some phenomenon (e.g., improved working conditions, increased employment, reduced domestic violence, safer food supply,

reduced stunting, improved national security, lower crime rate, reduced poverty, improved management of stock on a railway network).
- The way system components are organized or distributed, which can be physical (e.g., increased reach of internet infrastructure), biological (e.g., decreased deforestation, reduced atmospheric carbon) or social/institutional (e.g., increased financial market regulation).

Much of program design is about finding ways to influence the kinds of variables as just described.

The project aim can be expressed as the desire to modify some substantial aspect of the world at large; it is the *impact* of the program in Theory of Change terms. It may be predefined by the funder/developer. For example, an aim may be to reduce mortality among children under five years of age from malnutrition by 5% in region X by 2025. The aim is often associated with an impact that can only be achieved in the long term, which may be beyond the program's ceiling of accountability [237] (i.e., the program's causal reach), beyond which it cannot be expected to have direct influence.

Because impacts are often beyond the scope of current program activities, a program *objective* needs to be defined that is considered the reachable indicator of program success or progress toward the (longer-term) aim: it is the measurable criterion used to make a final determination of whether the desired impact is likely; it is the impact for which a program can be held accountable. For this reason, an objective needs to be SMART:

- Specific
- Measurable
- Attainable
- Realistic
- Time-bound

In some cases, this objective will couched in terms of behavior rather than any of the previously listed types of impact. This can be because behavior is often more easily measured and because the link between performance of the behavior and the longer-term or larger-scale Impact variables are already well-established in the literature, such that behavior change should be a good indicator that the program goal will be achieved.

In the case of SuperAmma (see Box 5.1), the program was set up to change handwashing behavior. Since the link between handwashing and diarrheal disease is already well established, it did not make sense to use scarce resources to measure health impacts. The same might be true of a vaccination program. Where vaccine efficacy has already been established, the important question for programs is how to ensure vaccine uptake, and this uptake behavior is what it is most useful to measure.

Box 5.1

BCD Example

SuperAmma Objective

The basic public health problem addressed by the SuperAmma program was to reduce diarrheal disease. The aim was defined to reduce diarrheal disease among children under five in a particular rural Indian population.

After much discussion among stakeholders, and with reference to the SMART criteria, the following statement of objective was agreed at the SuperAmma Framing process:

- To sustainably increase baseline levels of handwashing with soap (HWWS) after defecation and before eating by 50% in the adult rural Indian population around location X [kept anonymous for ethical reasons].

The aim obviously takes the target behavior (defined next) and elevates it, in this case, to target population level to provide an indicator, given that increased HWWS is known from the academic literature to be correlated with diarrheal disease reduction (the state of the world the program wishes to influence).

Behavior

Having expressed the aims and objectives of the program, the next step is to define the behavior to be changed (see Box 5.2). This is rarely a simple task, and it is often iterative. However, it is vital to define the precise behavior that the program

Box 5.2

BCD Example

SuperAmma Target Behavior Definition

As a consequence of having conducted many similar campaigns on handwashing, program personnel rather easily agreed on the following definition:

- HWWS by adult household members in the target population.

Based on indications of public health relevance from the published literature, as well as biological plausibility, the target handwashing behaviors were further refined to be those occuring after fecal contact (both own defecation events, as well as contact with child feces in the case of child carers) and before contact with food (including preparation and serving events). Note just how precise these definitions are in terms of who, when, and what.

wishes to change. (Note that behavior means what people will *do*, not what they will *say, think, feel,* or *know*.)

Criteria for identifying target behaviors include:

- *Causal significance.* There should be strong evidence that the selected behavior has an impact on the program goal.
- *Incidence.* The behavior should be enacted by a large enough group of people, and often enough, to influence the program objective.
- *Changeability.* It should be possible to perform the targeted behavior with the resources available (e.g., it would be unhelpful to promote the use of products that are not available in the market), and for the program to be able to influence this behavior using the means available.

Brain

Here the primary question is to determine what kind of psychological processes are responsible for producing the behavior. Is the behavior habitual? If so, what cues it? What are the key motives that might drive performance of the target (rather than current) behavior? What plans do people make to carry out the behavior and does this help actual performance? Further, for target behaviors that are regularly practiced, it is useful to think whether the behavior can be *made* habitual. If there are barriers that can be removed by modifying the environment (e.g., by providing technological support), then the Assess Team should think about how to motivate the target audience to undertake the desired changes to their own environments (see Box 5.3).

Box 5.3

BCD EXAMPLE

SUPERAMMA PSYCHOLOGY OF CHANGE HYPOTHESIS

HWWS is naturally motivated by feelings of disgust, but also by a need to care for children who are unlikely to wash hands for themselves. It is probably also important that HWWS becomes part of an individual's sense of identity to make sure it is sustainably practiced. Including HWWS as part of everyday manners—that is, behaviors engaged in to ensure that one doesn't pass any infections on to others (e.g., by shaking with dirty hands)—could also be motivating and be felt as a sense of social obligation.

Body

The primary target of the behavior change effort is those individuals whose behavior must change to achieve the desired impact. This may be a single individual (in the case of self-help programs) or institutions (such as the prison system), or it may include whole populations. The target group is labeled *body* in the Theory of Change because BCD emphasizes the situational and physical nature of behavior, which is always behavior by an individual interacting with their environment. But, of course, at a program level, measurements are taken at the population level, summing over individual cases. The typical demographic characteristics of the target individual—gender, age, education level—can be considered bodily traits and thus define a typical target population profile.

The more tightly defined the target group is, the easier it is to develop the program. To increase the chances of a healthy pregnancy, for example, should a public health program target all adolescents and young adults to set up good eating habits? Or would it be feasible to target just those women in the first months of pregnancy? Do mothers and husbands play an important role in deciding what pregnant women eat? Such people may form an important secondary target audience—as may teachers, social opinion leaders, or other key influencers. The more that can be learned about the target groups the better the program can influence them. Hence the need to gather together what is known about daily life, work patterns, education, and the social and physical infrastructures in which they live. (See Box 5.4.)

Environment (Touchpoints)

The environment is the place where program activities are implemented. For example, posters may be placed in public places or messages broadcast from loudspeakers on the tops of roving cars. These are considered the intervention's *touchpoints*, the places and times through which program activities come into contact with the target population. What are the ways in which they might experience the program? Do they currently have or watch TV or listen to the radio, and, if so, what programs do they enjoy? Do they wait at bus stops; use rickshaws;

Box 5.4

BCD Example

SuperAmma Target Population

In the framing process, the following was also agreed:

- Primary target: Mothers in the intervention area with children under five.
- Secondary target: Other carers of children, primary and elementary school teachers, and Gram Panchayat head.

Box 5.5

BCD EXAMPLE

SUPERAMMA TOUCHPOINTS ANALYSIS

The decision of the core team (even prior to the Framing process), given budgetary constraints and field logistics, was to deliver the campaign to individual villages, via a traveling pair of implementers conducting a series of activities over a relatively few days (so as to allow for the program to be scaled up). This suggested a program based on community-level activities (with street theater elements) as well as innovative media (such as animated cartoons). The approach was borrowed from the practice of Unilever's rural soap marketing practices in India.

---

attend village gatherings such as weddings, funerals, and political meetings; wait in line for water; or attend parent–teacher meetings? In the Assess step, data are gathered about the touchpoints where target populations can be contacted and affected; a more detailed consideration of what contact behavior settings look like, and their relevance, can only be determined once a more complete picture of what the campaign will look like has been developed (i.e., after the Create step). (See Box 5.5.)

Behavior Setting

Here, the interest is to isolate the contexts within which the target behaviors occur currently and potential intervention settings (which may be different from target behavior settings). In Part I, we learned that behavior settings have the following components: stages, roles, routines, scripts, motives, norms, infrastructure, and focal objects (props). These issues are typically not well understood by existing literature (which is seldom specific about the physical and social contexts of actual behavior as it is practiced); hence, at the Assess step, not much may be known about them. Nevertheless, insiders with knowledge of the target behaviors may be able to come up with some hypotheses as to the setting-related factors that may be determining behavior and how they might be changed.

Using this process, the Assess Team can produce ideas about what form they think the intervention itself should take. Interventions are the ideas, materials, and activities through which environments are modified (in the form of an implementation). What should the program promoter doing a household visit say and do? What should the poster at the bus stop say? These can be agreed as hypotheses to be tested in the field via formative research or even through simple small-scale prototyping prior to the Build step, if possible, to eliminate any ideas that obviously aren't going to work. Prototyping can be as simple as getting informants to tell stories about how the desired process could take place (e.g., how they would

Box 5.6

BCD EXAMPLE

SuperAmma BCD Checklist

SuperAmma Program

Factor	Subfactor	Now	Desired	Change strategy	Unknowns
State of the world	Aim	High diarrhea among children under five in India	Reduced diarrhea rates		Unlikely to be measurable
	Objective				
Behavior	Target	No soap use when handwashing	Regular soap use when handwashing		Best means of measuring HWWS
	Who	No one	Adults and children		
	When	Never	After defecation, handling child feces, and before eating		
	Where	No designated place	Close to household		
Environment	Physical				
	Biological	Contaminated environment		None	
	Social	Role models don't use soap	Role models use soap	Get prominent people to endorse soap use	
Brains	Executive	Everyone knows soap use is healthy already	Identity supermom	Change identity, not knowledge	
	Motivated	Smelly/greasy hands can prompt disgust; Mothers want status for their children	Even "clean" hands can be "dirty"; Ideal mothers HWWS	Disgust, Nurture, Affiliation to be emphasized	Which of these motives is most important lever of change for HWWS?

Body	Reactive	No HWWS habit	HWWS practiced without thinking	Bathroom stickers	How long does it take to form a habit?
	Traits	Conscientious, female			What other characteristics are important?
	Physiology Senses	Smelly/sticky/visibly dirty hands	More aware of dirty hands	Use Glo Germ™ demonstration	How to use at scale?
Behavior setting	Stage	Bathroom area in front of compound			Is change needed? Possible?
	Roles	Good-enough mom?	HWWS is mannerly behavior	Mothers teach good manners to their children	What other good manners are commonly taught?
	Routine	Handwashing with water only	Includes soap use		
	Script	Proper handwashing	Complete handwashing event includes soap use	Lots of examples of HWWS on display	
	Norms	No one does it	Others do it and expect me to do it too	Highlight "everyone thinks it is important to do it"	
	Props	Soap present	Handwash place established	Handwashing corner	How can practical difficulties be overcome?
	Infrastructure	Water source hard to access	Bowls/jugs in handwashing corner	Designate a handwashing corner	How can practical difficulties be overcome?

SuperAmma Program

	Touchpoints			
Intervention	Parent-teacher meetings, rickshaws, community meetings, Panchayat messenger	Community events, school events, posters on trees	Generate community buzz about importance of HWWS issue	What other kinds of events happen in villages?
Context		All deliver HWWS message?		
Programmatic	Rajiv Gandhi poverty reduction program, government vaccination programs, etc.			
Political	Hygiene competes with many other kinds of programs		Get government on board	How much can government be influenced?
Economic	Soap is perceived as expensive (but is not)		Reduce perceived cost of soap	
Social	Caste system influence on perceptions of "dirty" behavior?		Avoid any mention of caste	

HWWS = handwashing with soap.

go about acquiring the new product in question), getting them to role-play a new role (e.g., a supermom), or drawing a picture of an ideal family and then describing how it is different from existing examples. The result of these efforts of imagination and practice can be a first draft of the program's Theory of Change, as links have at this point been suggested from intervention to implementation, leading to brain-based change and, thence, to behavior change.

Intervention

With a set of touchpoints decided, the set of relevant behavior change techniques in hand, and other knowledge about the behavior setting available, ideas about an incipient Theory of Change can be developed, linking touchpoints to psychological changes to behavior change. More specifically, potential intervention components should first be matched to the useful qualities of possible touchpoints. For example, household visits are a likely site for in-depth social interaction, being private and narrowly focused, although not likely to involve multiple visits and, hence, not long-term. It may actually be the site where the target behavior is performed as well. This situation suggests use of one-on-one–based components such as peer interviews that try to facilitate barrier identification and problem-solving, advise target individuals about environmental restructuring or how to change routine, and perhaps induce a commitment from the client there and then.

On the other hand, bus stops are public places where the type of people visiting cannot be controlled or managed and visits may be repeated, but each visit is short in duration and attention may be focused elsewhere. So components such as posters that provide instructions on how to perform the behavior, emphasize the value of the desired choice, or suggest a substitute behavior are more likely to be effective in that situation.

Second, the question should be asked whether the mental change hypothesized to result from contact with that component is likely to have an effect on the target behavior in its setting. In the case of the household visit, is pledging to perform the behavior (a form of commitment) likely to influence actual performance if the target behavior typically takes place in the house? Could its effectiveness be supplemented by demonstration of the target behavior during the visit? In the case of the bus stop, would information about how to engage in performance of the target behavior be effective if the target behavior doesn't actually require much skill? Is the behavior to substitute for current practice obvious to everyone without much variation in opinion (so you can be sure of the consequence of the technique)?

Revaluation of the target behavior that results from exposure, attention, and mental processing can occur both at the point of exposure and over time, as individuals reflect on the surprising stimulus and continue to learn about it. The completed Revaluation can be considered the *output* of the intervention in Theory of Change terms.

Draft Theory of Change

Participants in the framing process thus endeavor to agree to the answers to the Theory of Change questions (as far as possible). Ensuring proper consideration of all factors that might determine behavior and about which something should be known can be facilitated by use of the BCD checklist (derived from the list of behavioral determinants in the Behavior Determination model discussed earlier). This tool helps to organize knowledge from the literature and the experts into a set of findings about what is known and unknown about the hypothesized mechanisms of change. The unknowns constitute the factors that require further research during the Build step (discussed next). The filled-in checklist is a useful summary record of the Assess step and provides the agenda for the next step, Build (see Box 5.6 for an example from the SuperAmma campaign). A second output should be a Formative Research Protocol that outlines the logistics and data collection methods for fieldwork with members of the target population, should additional data collection be required.

Build

The Build stage is designed to fill in any missing information in the developing Theory of Change. This typically involves primary data collection called formative research [238].

FORMATIVE RESEARCH

The purpose of formative research is to answer the questions that those in the framing process were unable to answer and to explore hypotheses about how to change the targeted behaviors (given the type of learning failure that seems to be responsible).

Behavior, as we have seen, is not just a function of rational decision-making but is also controlled by motives, which may be subconscious, and automatisms of which people are entirely unaware. It is also critically a function of behavior settings: the roles, scripts, stages, props, and social control that surround behavior. Therefore, formative research the Behavior Centered Design (BCD) way uses data collection techniques that focus on getting at an understanding of situated behavior. (A manual detailing how to implement the package of field methods developed to conduct BCD-style formative research is available on the Web.)

There are an endless number of techniques that can be used to study behavior and its determinants. One can participate in the lives of the target audience, film them, ask them to play a game online, use sensors to record what they do, tell them stories, ask them to create collages, or co-create products. How then can we decide which methods to use in a formative research study?

I argue that better data collection methods are more realistic. This can be defined quite precisely. First, the process of data collection can itself be seen as a situation, typically involving some form of social interaction (at minimum because researchers are present with a focal individual) [77]. This situation is typically quite different from that in which the target behavior takes place. Often, an interview is quite an artificial situation—that of a formalized social interaction in some location and time quite remote from performance of the target behavior, such as a lab room. Also, the behavior required of the informant is verbal behavior, which requires executive control to produce (i.e., it is thoughtful and consciously considered). If the target behavior, on the other hand, is produced automatically—for example, because it is habitual—then this is another way in which the behavior occurring during data collection is far from that actually under investigation. I consider data collected under circumstances closer to the conditions under which the behavior is normally produced to be of higher quality. This is because it is more likely to be accurate evidence of the processes that potentially need changing. (In an interview, a person can report that they regularly perform the behavior and that it is habitual to them when in fact they don't engage in the behavior at all. This is why self-report data are so often at odds with that resulting from observation.)

I therefore rank the kinds of data collection methods according to the type of behavior they require of the person providing the data and the relationship between the situation of the data collection event and that of the target setting. The best data collection methods are near, situationally and psychologically, to the behavior the program is trying to change. (For an example from the SupraAmma project, see Box 6.1.)

Box 6.1

BCD Example

SuperAmma Formative Research
Staff spent three weeks in rural Indian villages collecting data on existing and potential behavioral practices and related psychological and environmental factors, using the following methods:

- Video ethnographies of women with children under five, ensuring that all daily activities were filmed.
- Household water, sanitation, and hygiene facilities were inventoried, including all types of soap and its uses.
- Behavior trials, in which informant household members were urged to wash their hand with soap at relevant times of day and then visited several days later to see how well they fared.
- Key informant semistructured interviews to conduct the motives mapping, attribute ranking, and other projective exercises.

Near Techniques

Situated observation is the closest type of data collection, especially when it takes place with minimal interference by the observer. For example, in *participant observation*, the observer goes through the motions of performing the target behavior themselves, as well as trying to learn about how and when individuals from the target population perform the behavior. This method has a double focus, on self and other. The observer in this case also engages in performance to see what it feels like in their own body, as a further source of information about what it takes to engage in the behavior.

Video ethnography is a method that uses an individual close in their characteristics to those of the observed individual as the videographer (to minimize disruption). The idea is simply to follow someone from the target population around while they engage in normal daily activities, filming them as they do so, especially those behaviors of interest to the program.

On-site Prototyping or *Co-creation* is a more dynamic, active form of within-situation data collection. It involves program and target population members working together in situations as close to reality as possible, generating and/or testing ideas. These ideas can be about new designs for objects that can be used to facilitate the behavior, infrastructural manipulations to support performance of the target behavior, or purely behavioral insights and experimentation, such as improvised role play, to explore new routes and routines to achieve behavior setting goals.

Often experiments on each of these types of ideas can be conducted in parallel. In particular, use of a new object may require new types of action during role play or to be supported by infrastructural changes as well. For example, introducing a handwash stand to facilitate handwashing with soap requires that people accept new actions in the script for their handwashing routine: the use of soap. It also requires that water be provided on-site so that hands can be rinsed of soap and that soap itself (the object in this example) be present where needed.

Co-creation with members of the target population can begin with a minimum viable prototype (MVP) for each sort of modification to the setting. An MVP can consist of a very simple mock-up of a new object (e.g., some form of replacement for soap that achieves the same objective of removing pathogens from body surfaces), a random idea about a behavioral strategy to inject soap use into the handwashing routine (e.g., via storytelling about how to wash hands properly), or a low-cost, easy-to-install method for ensuring quick access to a water supply as an infrastructural support for the target behavior. These MVPs can then be elaborated as necessary and appropriate from testing on-site.

In-Between Methods

The in-between methods rely on data collected in situations that closely mimic the target behavior setting (e.g., being in the same place and time), but performance is explicitly requested by the observer, so it may not be representative of what the individual normally does. The investigator may ask the participant to do something that is not in their regular repertoire and for which they don't have the requisite skills, but which is—or bears some interesting relationship to—the target behavior. For example, just to see how they might try to manage performance, given more or less conducive circumstances, we may ask people to wash their hands with soap but with or without a ready source of water. Such data therefore have some ecological validity but are not as valid as more naturalistic observation.

Behavior trials and *behavior demonstrations* fall into this category. A behavior trial differs from a behavior demonstration in that the trial leaves the participant to engage in the target behavior over some period while on their own (with a follow-up to ask how they got on), while in a demonstration the requested behavior is observed in situ, with researchers present at the time of observation. I assume that because they are being watched and because the behavior may be unfamiliar that such demonstrations are produced quite consciously and normatively.

Far Methods

Most of the standard techniques used in social science research fall into this category, despite its low quality (given the BCD classification scheme). *Interviews* and *focus group discussions* are the techniques most often used in formative research but often are the most remote from the circumstances of actual behavior, since they are typically conducted in specialized, formal situations and demand consciously produced behavior (typically verbal responses to questions posed by the observer). Because they are so familiar, it isn't necessary to discuss them further here.

So-called projective techniques, developed primarily in consumer research, attempt to reduce one aspect of ecological invalidity: production by the wrong type of psychological control (i.e., executive control rather than motivational). They do this by trying to directly tap into motivated behavior production for behaviors that are normally produced in this fashion.

The BCD formative research toolkit contains many techniques that fall into this category. *Motive mapping*, for example, presents informants with a story-board of the target behavior (i.e., a set of drawings that depict the desired sequence of actions, properly situated for the informant's cultural group), followed by a story ending that depicts some form of reward being given (e.g., the depicted individual's spouse saying "I love you for doing that!"). The informant is then asked to indicate whether this kind of feedback or ending is realistic, likely, motivating, etc. Obviously, this method, despite the situational distance from its normal context, attempts to reduce psychological distance by simulating the behavioral context using a pictorial narrative and to minimize reflection by focusing directly on the reward from performance.

Attribute ranking puts a number of pictures or objects in front of the respondent and asks them to rank these stimuli from low to high on some dimension. For example, food items can be ranked according to how healthy or affordable they are, or pictured body types can be ranked on how ideal they are. (See the BCD Formative Research Protocol document, available on the web at https://www.lshtm.ac.uk/bcd, for many more examples.)

Other Methods

There is a type of data collection that doesn't readily fit this typology, as it doesn't require individuals to produce behavior at the time of data collection. Rather, it depends on the observer collecting information from indicators left in the environment produced as a *consequence* of performance. Here, the investigator is left picking up traces of what behavior has left behind. An example is trying to determine what someone has eaten by gathering food wrappers from their household garbage. This is obviously quite indirect and so again does not provide data of optimum quality from the BCD perspective.

BCD therefore suggests use of a variety of data collection methods and provides a decision-making criterion for selecting among them, prioritizing methods that capture real behavior in its proper setting. In the absence of these gold standard approaches, second-best methods of behavior trials, role-playing (preferably in the appropriate behavior setting), or simulation of some kind (i.e., imagined behavior on computers, projective techniques) should be preferred. Third-best are verbal reports (e.g., interviews, focus group discussions), historical case studies, or cultural similarities from other groups. In all cases, more interactive, iterative methods that involve participants as whole people in real situations should be preferred.

An additional choice criterion is often triangulation, or the use of several methods having a variety of strengths and weaknesses to study the same phenomenon. This can ensure that a more complete picture is obtained, assuming that certain aspects of a phenomenon will be better revealed by a method more specialized for viewing the world from that angle and that the biases inherent in use of any one method can be overcome in this way [239].

Hypothesis Testing

A good BCD investigator also brings theory to a field investigation. In every structured interaction during formative research the investigator should be looking at the problem through the eyes of the BCD categories set out in the checklist: what setting is this I am seeing, and what are its components, its purposes, and its history? How does the target behavior serve this setting and how could it make a setting more productive? What primary motives are at play and could new ones be added? How could the target behavior be made more rewarding? And could the target behavior become habitual?

In common with consumer research, formative research can be conducted with an eye for major insights, or information that sheds new and surprising light on why people do what they do. For example, during participatory exercises in Zambia, we realized that the preparation of oral rehydration salts was seen as a cooking task, so ingredients were never measured properly (i.e., inappropriate rules were applied from a cooking setting), and mothers stockpiled the free packets so as not to waste them (the Hoard motive). In Indonesia, video ethnography showed mothers chasing children down the street trying to feed them family meals. Closer investigation revealed that children were not hungry because they had been fed snacks just before meal time to keep them quiet; otherwise, mothers might be accused by neighbors of poor parenting (motives: Hunger/Affiliation).

A formative research investigation can be as long or as short as time and resources allow. For a small project, it might consist of one investigator spending a couple of days in the company of representatives of the target audience (e.g., doing visits to relevant sites, such as households, factories, markets—wherever relevant behaviors are likely to be actually practiced—to observe and/or record behavior as well as collect other related data). If one is preparing a major project, however, weeks of more thorough investigation by a larger team might be warranted. In any case, the field team seeks to ensure sufficient knowledge is gained about the gaps in the BCD checklist. A rough guide might be to spend 5 to 10 percent of the total budget on the Build step.

DESIGN PROCESS

The next part of the Build step is to convert the findings of formative research into a Theory of Change for the program. I have broken down this process into nine steps (listed in Box 6.2), which take the process from a large number of findings derived from the field to production of a creative brief that reflects a single program focus. These steps are best achieved using a team with a variety of expertise

---

Box 6.2

BCD Tool

Program Design Process Steps
1. Download significant *findings* using an organizing *framework*.
2. Cluster Findings into *Themes* (i.e., rich areas for exploration) using *expert consensus*.
3. Brainstorm *Ideas* that address target behavior via Theme using *analogies*.
4. Build *Platforms* from (promising) Ideas, incorporating related findings, Themes, and additional knowledge using *clustering*.
5. Perform *Appraisal* by ranking Platforms using *Platform assessment criteria*.
6. Agree program *focus* using stakeholder *decision-making*.
7. Develop program *Components* using *expert consensus*.
8. Agree to Program *Theory of Change* using stakeholder *decision-making*.
9. Write *Briefs* (defining task based on focus and [set of] Touchpoints) for Creative/Delivery/Evaluation Agencies using *forms*.

---

and degrees of acquaintance with the program problem and population. Getting the relevant people (from a variety of stakeholder groups) to work together in a workshop is often an optimal solution to identify the best program focus [240].

Once the formative research data have been analyzed, program managers are in position to identify the causal links that they believe are most likely to have a significant influence on making the target population perform the target behavior. This part of the process remains more art than science, but development of a complete Theory of Change helps to isolate specific causal links that are currently missing in the target population's way of life but that, if introduced, would have a large impact on the likelihood of the target behavior being widely practiced.

Getting Some Focus

The Program Design problem that arises at this point can be seen as one of shrinking the mass of information produced by the Build step into a single insight that forms the foundation of the program focus. To achieve this, I follow a process that is as standardized as possible, given the mercurial nature of creativity. Many of the steps in this process can be described as examples of conceptual blending (see Box 6.3), in which a concept cluster of a certain size is added to or subtracted

---

Box 6.3

BCD Theory

Conceptual Blending
The steps in which concepts are aggregated (i.e., Steps 2, 3, 4, and 6) can be viewed as examples of conceptual blending. Conceptual blending is a theory developed originally in linguistics but subsequently applied in a variety of fields to describe processes of abstraction and creativity [241–244].

Conceptual blending involves making comparisons between several different conceptual domains. It takes place through three steps:

- Recognize an analogy between concept Domain 1 and Domain 2 (called input spaces in the previous diagram). This produces a mental mapping of some of the elements of Domain 1 into Domain 2, and vice versa.
- Recognize the elements of Domain 1 and 2 that are held in common as a set that can form the foundation of a generic space (a third conceptual domain generated by this process of blending). This abstraction can serve as one of the grounds for further mental elaboration in later steps.
- Build Domain 3 (the blended model) in a separate mental space, from the analogical elements of Domains 1 and 2, but also adding in relevant background knowledge so that the new domain has emergent characteristics of its own (what conceptual blending practitioners call a *conceptual integration network* [246]).

A classic example is trashcan basketball [247]. Imagine the Creative Team is sitting around trying to come up with Themes by writing down phrases on pieces of paper. Some of these ideas are immediately discounted, and the paper thrown into a trashcan. One of the team calls out "Goal!" This exclamation is based on an insight—an understanding that an object in one conceptual space (i.e., a wad of paper) corresponds to an object in another space (a large leather ball in the mental cluster that describes the game of basketball). The crumpled-up piece of paper thus becomes a ball—exploiting a mapping between two conceptual domains. This sparks a process that results in a whole system of correspondences between the two domains of "throwing away waste" and "basketball game." These mental space connections can be based on identity, similarity, or analogy. The paper-wad-as-ball is based on similarity (both objects are round) and analogy (throwing into a trashcan is like throwing into a basket).

Because it is based on only partial mappings from the source domains, plus independently added material, the blended space (trashcan basketball) has a unique representational structure of its own—that is, it has emergent qualities that can be exploited (e.g., which might be surprising). For example, the realization that one can add meaning to throwing away a piece of paper by turning it into an act of skill development or even a competitive game is a novel idea that can be inspiring.

Conceptual blending forms the foundation of the creative process in BCD, as each of the most difficult steps—those of generating more complex concepts—can be seen as building up connections into a more complex concept using this mechanism. From this theoretical perspective, Themes, Ideas, Platforms and Foci are simply increasingly complex concept clusters formed by taking the blended domain from one step and then building upon it by adding elements from other source domains as well as additional background knowledge into a larger blended domain. The links to even more abstract concepts might be made using mappings from the generic space to a new source domain to create the new blended domain. In this way, hierarchical relationships can be established, drawing in mental resources from increasingly disparate conceptual domains. The process finally results in the most robust conceptual cluster, called a focus. The Creative Team then selects from among alternative potential Foci in the final step prior to writing the creative brief with the chosen focus as its central message.

---

from to form a related cluster of a different size. A number of tricks can be used to help groups go through these steps of conceptual blending, such as having a clear goal, enforcing equality among participants, complete concentration (to achieve a flow state), close listening (without criticism), relying on familiarity rather than formality, and maximizing communication to achieve the most productive levels of cooperation [240].

Getting to a campaign focus is achieved step-wise. Step 1 is to get all the salient findings into the mix. This is facilitated by introducing an organizing framework to stimulate knowledge that might otherwise get forgotten and to organize what is likely to be a large quantity of material. This can be achieved by summarizing important points from existing knowledge and formative research on Post-it notes, which are put on a wall for all to see. This is most quickly and effectively achieved by having everyone present (who should represent all major stakeholder groups) individually produce findings by brainstorming during the workshop.

The categories in the BCD checklist can be used to organize these findings. Findings can relate to anything from the checklist: traits of the target population, their motivations, habits, socioeconomic level, kinds of major investments they make, characteristics of their social networks, religious beliefs, etc. In this discussion, I will use an example from a recent maternal nutrition program in Indonesia to illustrate the kinds of results that arise from each step of Program Design. In this program, one finding was "Offspring are expected to send a significant proportion of earnings from their first job back to their parents." These snippets of knowledge are then grouped according to some common element (Step 2). This, and subsequent clustering steps, are most quickly and effectively achieved through group-think—basically having everyone go about the room moving stickies with some common element together into clusters. Each cluster, representing a common thread, is given a name and becomes a Theme. In our example, a number of findings were related to the Theme of "Indonesian mothers are thrifty." (For example, we determined from a cluster of findings that it is seen as virtuous to husband family resources and to save for a rainy day.)

Once all the findings have been organized into Themes, the Themes are themselves augmented with additional bits of supporting knowledge and creative insight from the assembled group (often based on making some analogy between conceptual domains) into Ideas (Step 3). One of our nutritional Ideas (related to the previous Theme) was "Make eating while pregnant into an investment" (because a fetus is an investment in the family's future). A number of candidate Ideas should result from this process of repeated aggregation. (Other Ideas included the insight that Indonesians are "not big on big"—they are worried that at term their fetus might be too big to be delivered naturally and inexpensively—and that the moment when new wives learn how to cook for their husbands was a teachable moment).

These Ideas must then be built up into potential Platforms, or complex concepts, that can support the program as a whole (Step 4). Our nutritional Platform that built on the investment Idea was "Babies are the investment with the highest return available to target households." This is getting closer to an organized cluster of knowledge and insight that could motivate behavior change. Several Platforms should be developed through this developmental process.

At this point, it is necessary to identify a single conceptual framework with which to move forward into the Create step. To determine which Platform has the "longest legs," each is subjected to group appraisal using several (rather subjective) Platform Assessment Criteria (Step 5):

- *Richness*: the number of associations which can be conceptually linked to the basic premise.

- *Cogency:* the tightness of causal links it introduces and, hence, the likelihood that it will change the target behavior.
- *Plasticity:* the degree to which the Platform addresses a modifiable determinant of the target behavior.
- *Novelty:* the level of surprise it should inspire.
- *Defensibility:* the degree to which other agents/campaigns are incapable of making the same claims.
- *Acceptability:* the degree to which the platform is acceptable to the target population.

Grids of two the most important dimensions (e.g., finding those Platforms that are expected to be both rich and acceptable) or summed rankings on all of these criteria can be used for this weighting process. When making this ranking in Indonesia, the investment-based Platform was determined to be the best for our nutritional program.

However, Platforms are often still abstract and may not be directly related to the target behaviors (i.e., they can still relate to other aspects of life). They therefore require additional focus, which again typically requires a bit of creative insight (Step 6). To continue with our example, the focus arrived at was "Consuming the target foods is the best investment in the household's best investment: a (financially/socially) successful offspring."

The chosen focus should then form the basis for the brief that goes to the Creative Agency/Team as the organizing principle for the development of the intervention itself.

Obviously, a major consideration is whether the chosen focus will pass the Theory of Change test—that is, it should be surprising, cause revaluation of the target behavior (e.g., by adding value in the form of new associated motives), and help cause performance as well. If it does not do so satisfactorily, it has to be modified through further creative effort so that it will. How this can be achieved is discussed further in the following text, but the initial choice of focus should nevertheless be checked for plausibility with respect to a draft Theory of Change at this point. For example, it can be field-tested with a small sample to determine whether it has real potential. If not, then modifications should be made. (See Box 6.4 for an example from the SuperAmma project.)

Component Development

However, the Design Process is not yet complete. The basic kinds of program components need to be determined (Step 7). Overall program design can be said to depend upon a single criterion: finding the mix of components that are likely to have the maximum combined effect in terms of behavior change and that will produce the maximum impact (i.e., biggest change in program objective) for a given budget. In short, this means finding the components that, per dollar, most strongly flow through the Theory of Change mechanisms, disrupting the

Box 6.4

BCD Example

SuperAmma Focus

Handwashing with soap can become habitual if inculcated early in life and thus produce sustained behavior change. The task of producing this kind of inculcation lies with the primary child carer: the mother. In rural India, the identity for women with greatest social importance lies is in being good mothers (i.e., in being good at Nurture). Hence, the focus is

> Very good mothers—supermothers—are those who instill hygienic habits, particularly handwashing with soap, in their offspring (e.g., via calling them "good manners"—a reference to the Disgust motive).

This focus thus encompasses several added motives (including Status, or social aspiration, and Disgust) to the basic identity of a mother (associated with the primary domain motive, Nurture) in this population and links performance of this identity specifically to the target behavior of handwashing with soap. The SuperAmma concept hints at mothers as superheroes, who have the job of not just being caretakers but teachers of the next generation. In this way, it also provides a specific mechanism for ensuring that the practice can spread, as parenting strategies can be mimicked, and will be automatically replicated in the next generation.

Contact Setting (where people come into contact with the components) in ways that work through to the Target Behavior Setting (where behavior change must happen). The question is how to know what combinations of components are most synergistic. Unfortunately, little is known about this, so much remains guesswork.

Why do I think that using multiple components, each with a different causal pathway, is better than relying on a single one, given whatever power each might have? Most programs seem loath to depend exclusively on, for example, just using mass media. This may be due to fears that "putting all one's eggs in a single basket" is risky, given the considerable unknowns that usually prevail in terms of whether the postulated Theory of Change is correct. In most cases, it seems sensible to spread the risk across several causal pathways.

So, while the focus can be thought of as the central message to be communicated, programs are typically not just about delivering a single message in a single way, but rather rely upon multiple channels of delivery. At this stage, the basic kinds of intervention components to be undertaken should be determined.

The components of an intervention can be classified by the particular combination of touchpoint, activity, channel, and behavior change technique (BCT) they utilize (see Table 6.1). I will call these the *facets* of a component.

Table 6.1. FACETS OF INTERVENTION COMPONENTS

Facet	Feature	Theory of Change Element	Examples
Touchpoint	Time/place	Environment	Household living room in the evening, Saturday food market, Sunday morning religious service
Activity	Situation or context	Behavior setting	Demonstration/simulation of target behavior, persuasive face-to-face interaction, interactive game, educational lecture, community event
Channel	Information transmission modality	Body	Radio (aural), TV (visual + aural), physical therapy (tactile)
Behavior Change Technique	Psychological mechanism	Brain	Verbal persuasion about capability, emotional social support, adding object to environment, social comparison

Touchpoints are essentially the place and time at which the intervention will be delivered. For example, people can be reached in their living rooms at night, while shopping at the food market, or while waiting for a train at the station.

Second, activities are situations within which to convey the information (if one is depending on messaging) or of placing the environmental modification (if that is the component), making particular reference to the most relevant aspects of the behavior setting. Thus, community events can be created specific to the campaign—situations in which a location is taken over, specialized equipment may be set up (e.g., for a music concert or film display), and unusual behaviors performed (e.g., dancing, singing). On the other hand, the activity/situation may be a regular, everyday context such as a waiting for the bus to work every weekday morning at the bus stop in which nothing out of the ordinary occurs except the appearance of a new poster on a nearby wall.

BCD is particularly associated with a particular kind of activity: emo-demos (short for "emotional demonstrations"). These are activities, often participatory, which are inexpensive to produce, take only a short time to enact, can involve numerous participants, and align with program objectives. Their core function is to cause an emotional "Aha!" moment—that is, they seek to produce a memorable experience, likely to be recalled later in a way that will spark performance of the target behavior. For example, to promote exclusive breastfeeding, young mothers are shown what the tummy of their baby would look like if they were not exclusively breastfed. First, milk alone is put into a transparent plastic bag, and mothers are invited to drink this, which they readily do. However, they are then asked what else they feed their babies, and these foods are then added to the bag (e.g., crisps, snacks), creating a disgusting-looking mess. When asked if they will drink this, they refuse, and are told that nevertheless, this is what they are asking their babies to eat. This produces a revelation that leads to new feeding practices.

Third, the channel is the means by which information (or a new reward or punishment) will be passed to the intended audience. For example, people can be reached in their living rooms via TV broadcast, at the market by a product display or demonstration, or in a train station via a billboard or poster. Determining the most profitable mix of components can be aided by information about who in the target population makes use of the various channels of communication (e.g., TV, radio, newspaper, mobile phone messaging, etc.). Data concerning the reach of various channels can often be purchased from media monitoring companies. When the task isn't to message to the target population, the channel can also simply be the component itself, such as a speed bump in the road or fluoride added to a water supply.

Finally, a BCT specifies the psychological mechanism by which a particular determinant of behavior is expected to be influenced (and, hence, contribute to behavior change). Several quite different taxonomies are available. The first, produced by Susan Michie and colleagues, was derived through expert consensus, based on a large literature search in health psychology and related fields; it identifies a very large number of BCTs (over 120 at last count) in 16 different categories, such as goals and planning, comparison of outcomes, identity, and social support [248]. Goal-setting, action planning, and commitment are example BCTs in the goals and planning category.

Gerjo Kok and colleagues have also produced a categorization, designed to be easy to comprehend and apply by behavior change programmers [249]. As a consequence, it includes categories such as Methods to Change Social Norms; Methods to Change Awareness and Risk Perception; Methods to Change Skills, Capability, and Self-Efficacy and to Overcome Barriers, and Methods to Change Organizations. Particular BCTs can fall into several of these categories.

A taxonomy closely aligned to BCD was suggested by Rik Crutzen and Gjalt-Jorn Ygram Peters [250] and is based in evolutionary theory (indeed, its BCTs come from a previous book by me and Val Curtis [96]). Crutzen and Peters call this set of BCTs "evolutionary learning processes." The number of such processes is relatively small and, as the name suggests, distinguishes different forms of learning that can result from exposure to a particular component of an intervention. Example evolutionary learning processes range from the simplest (and first-evolved) mechanism, habituation/sensitization, to the most complex (and last-evolved), reflective learning/autobiographical memory. For example, habituation can be expected to occur from repeated exposure to a simple environmental modification, such as a speed bump in the road, while Reflective learning might result from hearing a narrative about what happened to someone else in a similar situation (e.g., during a one-on-one therapeutic interview).

Which system of BCTs you wish to use is a personal choice, but potential BCTs should be matched to the combined qualities of the touchpoints, activities, and channels already chosen. For example, household visits are a likely site for in-depth social interaction, being private and narrowly focused, although not likely to involve multiple visits and, hence, not long-term. It may actually be the site where the target behavior is performed as well. This situation suggests use of one on one based techniques such as

- Facilitate barrier identification and problem-solving.
- Advise on environmental restructuring.
- Change routine.
- Prompt commitment from the client there and then.
- Elicit and answer questions.

On the other hand, bus stops are public places where the type of people visiting cannot be controlled or managed and visits may be repeated, but each visit is short in duration and attention may be focused elsewhere. So techniques such as the following should be appropriate in this case:

- Provide instruction on how to perform the behavior.
- Emphasize choice.
- Prompt self-recording.
- Suggest behavior substitution.

Thus, some activities can't be delivered via certain kinds of channel: for example, large community events can't depend on one-to-one contact with target popula-tion members. Similarly, static media like billboards must be used very creatively indeed to convey certain kinds of BCTs, such as self-talk (provoking people to provide commentary on their own performance of the target behavior) or re-warding completion of the target behavior.

Thus, one component of a campaign might be a mass media broadcast. In this case, the touchpoint is the household at night, the activity is the everyday before-bed routine/setting, the channel is a television broadcast, and the BCT might be demonstrating approval by important social others. The market demonstration has a touchpoint of town marketplace on Saturday afternoon, the activity of the weekly food shop, the channel of narrative dramatization (a skit), and BCT of stimulating anticipation of future rewards. The billboard has the touchpoint of a particular platform at the bus stop whenever the target individual happens to be waiting for the bus; the activity is waiting for the bus, the channel is printed matter, and the BCT conveys new, unexpected consequences of performing an undesirable behavior. To these components, the campaign committee might add an emo-demo at a community event and a group pledge (touchpoint of commu-nity event, activity of face-to-face-interaction, channel of interpersonal verbal di-alogue, and BCT of agreeing a behavioral contract).

Decisions about each of the facets of a component are interdependent—that is, they should be complementary in terms of their ability to make each component, as delivered, maximally effective with respect to changing behavior in synergy with all the others.

Components should also be linked directly to the Theory of Change: touchpoints are particular points (and times) in the target population's lifestyle or routine; the activity is the type of situation or behavior setting in which the touchpoint becomes relevant, with particular emphasis on the role it requires the target population member to play (e.g., passive message recipient when reading a billboard vs. active participant in a pledging ceremony at a community event). The channel is the means by which the content of the activity is communicated to the body (e.g., via spoken message or visual modeling of the target behavior), and the BCT is the means by which a brain-based change is caused. Together, these contacts should produce behavior change as a consequence. Failures of a component to achieve each of these links can be assessed by the process evaluation, discussed later.

Thinking about components as combinations of these four facets (touchpoint, activity, channel, and BCT) helps to make it clear how they will work, which assists with the final task the Design Process participants have to complete: to develop a draft Theory of Change (Step 8). It is the job of the Theory of Change to provide a complete picture of the causes of the target behaviors and links to the impact and of formative research to ensure that all relevant aspects are known in sufficient, situated detail to inform intervention design, which is the next step (Create).

Draft Theory of Change and Campaign Analysis

Completing the Theory of Change requires thinking about how the focus will work itself through the various stages of outputs, outcomes, and impact to achieve program objectives. Box 6.5 shows the logical links that were agreed upon at this stage of program development by the SuperAmma program managers. Note that the Theory of Change is explicit about each subtask: how components will be *exposed* to the target population, get their *attention*, cause them to *process* the stimulus in ways that *add value* to the target behavior, increase *opportunities* for performance of the target behavior, and get it actually *selected* when those opportunities arise. Many components can work in roughly the same way, via the same mechanisms of psychological and behavioral change. On the other hand, some components may have specific roles in the overall plan: for example, teaser posters (which include only vague indicators of something about to happen) can work simply to attract attention to the campaign (i.e., achieve a degree of surprise), without causing further change (i.e., no revaluation or performance). Other components may rely on one specific mechanism to change one of the target behaviors (e.g., the SuperAmma skit was strictly about inducing disgust at having not washed hands before eating). It is the overall plan that must be balanced in the sense of ensuring that all those exposed to some likely combination of components will be

Box 6.5

BCD Example

SuperAmma Draft Theory of Change

This is the first draft of a Theory of Change diagram for the basic components of the program.

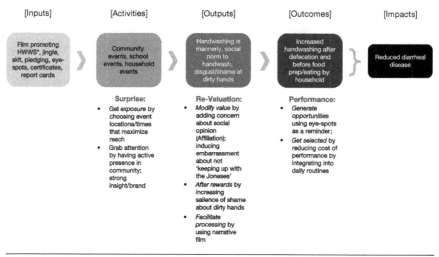

able to progress all the way to the end of the causal chain and change their behavior appropriately.

Development of such a complex framework should be helped by an ability to critique the overall design of the campaign. The tool in Box 6.6 can help think through this problem of complementarity for an imaginary program with a number of quite different components. Notice that it isn't expected that each component will help with all elements of the behavior change challenge—that is, achieve *Surprise, Revaluation,* and *Performance* alone. Nor will each component reach the entire target population (primary or secondary). It is for reasons like this that one must think through whether the intervention as a whole will likely achieve its aim.

BCD provides a second tool for this task as well (see Box 6.6), with specific criteria for determining whether the suite of proposed components should be considered as part of the program. Obviously, only components with strong causal links in the Theory of Change and that can be economically influenced by means available to the program should be considered. Further, only a limited number of components should be prioritized, as multiple elements tend to rapidly dissipate the power of an intervention. Also, complex interventions are harder to implement and evaluate. For all of these reasons, it is desirable for programs to focus on a very small number of behaviors and to use a unified, or branded (i.e.,

Box 6.6

BCD Tool

Intervention Component Analysis Tool

| | Components | | | | | |
Characteristics	Teaser Poster	Radio Drama	Television Ad	School Skit	Bathroom Reminder Stickers	Primary Health-Care Delivery Package
Primary segment 1 (women)	X	X	X		X	X
Secondary segment 2 (children)				X	X	
Exposure range	High	High	Low	Moderate	Moderate	Low
Exposure dosage	Moderate	Moderate	Low	Low	Moderate	Low
Surprise	X	X	X	X		
Revaluation		X	X	X		X
Performance					X	X
Delivery fidelity	High	High	High	low	Moderate	High
Delivery complexity	Moderate	Low	Low	High	Low	Moderate
Cost	High	High	High	High	Moderate	Moderate

easily identifiable), intervention campaign to address them. It is one of the jobs of the creative team to find a way to link the causal changes into a single carrier-wave idea that will become the central platform of the campaign.

The structure of the campaign thus should have a number of characteristics to be successful. These are listed in Box 6.7, which can be used to score potential designs against one another. Obviously, some variables in the Campaign Design Analysis Tool will be difficult to analyze at this early stage of program development (e.g., sustainability, cost-effectiveness). However, even rough estimates of the quality of the campaign with respect to these features should enable better decision-making about the overall look and feel of the proposed campaign. Again, branding should be considered as a factor, especially in noisy environments, to ensure that the campaign has an identity that distinguishes it.[1]

Box 6.7

BCD Tool

CAMPAIGN DESIGN ANALYSIS TOOL

Simplicity
[All campaigns have limited resources, the effect of which is diluted the more complex the communications/activities become.]

Measured by number of types of touchpoints, multiplied by number of components delivered per touchpoint, multiplied by number of target behaviors (higher values are worse).

Creativity/Branding
Ensure stakeholders agree a central identity (or unique selling point) for the campaign. (This is especially necessary for complex campaigns, or those which take place in a crowded messaging environment.) This allows all contacts with the target population to be branded in a way that

- Adds certainty about the source of the communication.
- Adds authority established by that source.
- Enables potential synergies between the content of those contacts.

Deliverability
- Corruptibility[a] (i.e., susceptibility to poor fidelity between planned intervention and implementation)
- Logistical complexity[a]
- Cost per exposure[a]
- Dependence on agents external to campaign

Evaluability
Ensure component delivery and impact can be readily monitored and evaluated so that (program level) learning can take place; this can depend on

- Ability to identify and monitor indicators (measurable variables) that the Theory of Change mechanisms have worked.
- Randomization of exposure to campaign components.
- Inclusion of control condition/population.
- Coverage (i.e., ensure number of recipients and numbers of contacts per recipient will be sufficient to reach desired impact).
- Identifiable consequences of program activities (e.g., compared to other, similar campaigns; related to branding).

Sustainability
Use methods that ensure activities can continue without further injections of time/money/staff from the program (e.g., institutionalize the activities)

Cost-Effectiveness
Measure of (expected) impact versus campaign cost

Context
Minimize dependence of impact on uncontrollable macro-environmental conditions or processes, including

- Activities of competing campaigns.
- General economic conditions.
- Involvement of extra-campaign agents playing central roles (e.g., village head, health professionals).
- Development, sales or distribution of program-specific products/services/technologies.

Scoring: Single point for each positive response; higher scores are better.
[a]Variable measured on dimension of low/high (with low getting the point).

Contextual factors are those that try to insulate the campaign from external influences that might reduce program effectiveness such as dependence on organizations outside the control of the program or disruptive economic conditions.

Effectiveness is also dependent on being able to deliver the components with good fidelity—otherwise the message or intended influence can be diluted or perverted. Sustainability is an important criterion in many cases because it takes time—for habits to form or for secondary processes to take place (e.g., buzz effects)—before maximum impact can be felt.

Creative Brief

With the components of the program now chosen (based on the Campaign Design Analysis Tool) and organized into a draft Theory of Change, the final task of the Design Team—or those on the Core Team responsible for development of the intervention materials—is to write a brief for a creative agency (Step 9). This brief is where all the critical information that those involved in designing the intervention must know. It is infused with behavioral information and insights because it has been arrived at through a rigorous process. It is the pivot that the project

Box 6.8

BCD Example

SuperAmma Creative Brief

1. Stakeholders
   - Project stakeholders are St. John's Research Institute (logistics coordinator), Centre of Gravity (creative agency), Mudra Max (rural activation agency), the London School of Hygiene and Tropical Medicine (project lead).
2. Background information
   - What are the facts about diarrhea and behavior change?
   - Diarrhea is endemic among children under five in the target population.
   - These women's lives are incredibly busy and their behavior tends to be rigidly bound in by their energetic, temporal social, and other requirements.
   - The most important behavior for reducing diarrhea is handwashing with soap.
   - What do we know about the target behaviors now?
   - Almost no one practices them currently.
3. Aim
   - We want to reduce diarrhea among children under five in peri-urban and rural low-income households in our pilot areas. This means changing the following behaviors among their caregivers: handwashing with soap after defecation and any contact with food.
4. Objective
   - Handwashing with soap after defecation and during food preparation among target profile individuals should increase at least 50 percent from baseline and be sustained for a period of at least six months.
5. Focus
   - Very good mothers are those who instill hygienic habits, particularly handwashing with soap, in their offspring.
6. Intervention design principles
   - Must work for rural and peri-urban settings and be scalable for the rest of India.
   - All implementation must work for low and no literacy communities.
   - Must be consistent with Theory of Change (i.e., including insight mechanisms of disgust, aspirational elicitation, remodeling of "good mother" role).
   - No mention of health or nutrition.
   - No knowledge transmission: film should communicate through common understandings, story arc, and feelings, not lecturing.
   - Tone: naturalistic.
   - Must demonstrate target behavior.
   - Must show benefit/consequence.

7. Agency deliverables and requirements
   - The core agency outputs will be a 10-minute animated film, scripted for disgust-based play; materials for pledging (e.g., certificate, eyespots); logistics plan for implementation in each village.
8. Budget and timeline
   - Not included here.

---

turns on moving from gathering and analyzing information to creating a behavior changing intervention. The brief should also contain essential information about the budget available for intervention and any constraints on the type of channel that can be used and time to project completion (see the Box 6.8).

The Build team may also write a report summarizing the findings of the formative research for publication or further use.

7

Create

The job of the Create step is to produce the materials that will go into the intervention. These materials have to be able to instigate the change mechanisms postulated in the Theory of Change. This will normally require that the creative *insight* (a surprising concept associated with the focus in the brief) be converted into an *intervention* (creative materials) and then into the *implementation* (environmental modification, through activities). This means it should cause surprise, which will, in turn, cause reinforcement learning that results in the choice of the target behavior as the best performance option. The learning strategy should also reflect which type of learning failure has been identified as responsible for the problem in the first place (e.g., super-stimulating object use or rare side-effects; see Table 1.2).

The strategy for causing Revaluation—hyping the evolved motive associated with the target behavior and/or adding or subtracting other motives—should also reflect the learning failure type. Ensuring that the Target Setting will facilitate Performance should also be considered as part of the creative brief. The process for getting to an actual intervention is described in the Box 7.1. It essentially expands out the program focus (resulting from the Design Process) into the suite of materials that will go into the intervention.

CREATIVE PROCESS

The Create step is primarily about the development of creative materials that form the components of the intervention (including implementation plans).

Box 7.1

BCD Tool

Create Process Description

1. Develop component *Content* using *imagination.*
2. Vet creative *Reverts* using *Component and Campaign Analysis tools.*
3. Pretest campaign *Components* using *behavior trials.*
4. Produce program *Materials* using *production processes.*

Developing component content is largely an imaginative exercise and so should be done by experts where possible. There are many types of creative agency from international conglomerates with a huge range of experts on tap to "barefoot" creatives, who might be local theater directors, artists, or entrepreneurs. Big international agencies will have experience of delivering not just "above the line" components (i.e., TV commercials, Internet content, billboards, etc.), but also "below the line" components (i.e., direct consumer contacts such as events in stores, football games in the community, etc.).

Briefing and managing a creative agency requires particular skills. For tips about how to conduct this relationship, see the Box 7.2.

Box 7.2

BCD Tool

Tips for Hiring/Managing a Creative Agency

Selecting an Agency
- Make a shortlist.
- Look at previous work: is it surprising, different?
- Meet the team: are they good listeners?
- Ask for a presentation; ask to see commercial and noncommercial work.
- Ask how strong the team is (sometimes you'll meet their star creative at this stage, but they'll never work on your campaign).
- If you ask for the team that works on commercial projects not charity projects, you may get a tougher, more professional job.
- Discuss behavior change with them; give them this monograph and ask for their thoughts
- Decide if they seem ready to flex and adapt to what you want.
- Figure out procurement: it can be hard to use public money to hire a creative agency; there may be a long tendering process that you have to build into your timeline.
- Recognize that creativity costs money; few agencies will be prepared to work pro bono (although some may have access to sources of subsidy for charity projects).

Briefing
- If you want something new and edgy, then your briefing should mirror this.
- Try briefing the agency on-site.
- Explain why what you are doing matters and the sort of exposure you might be able to get for them.
- Show them examples of the sort of campaign you like.
- If you make the process fun, exciting, and encouraging of wild ideas, you will motivate them.

- At the same time, set out the constraints, about budget, channels, tone.
- It's tempting to give a loose brief in the hope that the agency will come up with something magical that you haven't thought of. This rarely happens—creativity is stimulated by tight constraints, so stick to the brief throughout.

Reverts
- Once they've been briefed, the agency will expect to go away and come up with some ideas.
- When they come back, you may hate what they've done but try to stay positive: tell them what you like and why. When you really do like what they've done, convey your excitement.
- Prepare for multiple reverts in your timeline; you may be talking to your agency for months before they get it right.
- Use the toolbox in Box 7.3 to evaluate candidate ideas.
- At the end of each revert, summarize what you've agreed on. Try very hard not to go back on those agreements; otherwise, the agency can't progress
- If possible, try out agreed directions on the target audience; use prototypes of messages, products, or services so that you can "fail early and often."

Long Term
- When you've built a good relationship with a creative agency, try to use them again.

Having given the Creative Agency/Team their brief and some time, they will be expected to come back to the Core Team with their first set of ideas. The first reverts to the Core Team in these Creative Meetings will be in the form of potential concepts for the central focus of the campaign. Rarely will the first ideas brought back by the creative agency be powerful, on-brief, and acceptable to the client. Typically, several iterations of critique and revision will be required (Step 2). The idea is to use the criteria in the Behavior Centered Design (BCD) Component Analysis tool (see Box 7.3) to make this process more explicit and productive for each potential campaign component.

This tool includes novel elements specific to BCD. These elements are related to the Setting Transfer Problem (discussed earlier), or the fact that the setting in which contact with the program intervention takes place is rarely the same setting in which the target behavior itself will take place. The point is that it can be difficult both for individuals to hold intentions or memories from one setting (in which they become familiar with the campaign message) to another (in which they need to perform the target behavior), much less interpret a communication that places the imagination in yet another setting (e.g., depicted in some advertising narrative). To illustrate these differences, consider that a campaign using TV ads can have a contact setting of a target individual's living room at night (while they are watching TV). The TV ad comes on and depicts an elegant woman eating in a fancy restaurant (the Communication Setting). Meanwhile, the Target Setting (where the

Box 7.3

BCD Tool

Component Analysis Tool

Setting-Based

[The following aspects of settings should be scored with respect to two comparisons: Touchpoint vs. Target settings and Communication vs. Target settings; one point is scored per small (cognitive) difference between the element in the two settings.]

- Behavior's *stage*
- *Time delay* between exposure and performance of target behavior in the two settings
- Primary *actor*
- Primary actor's *role*
- Primary actor's primary *motive*
- Primary target's *routine*
- New *infrastructural support* for target behavior (suggested or provided)
- New *synomorphic support* for target behavior (suggested or provided)

Brand-Based

- Specific *brand elements* included
- Consistent with *brand aesthetics/feel/tone*
- *Uniqueness* of proposition/insight (a previously unknown, unrecognized, or underappreciated link between the target behavior and some value)
- *Defensibility*, or the ability to ensure that others can't copy the "active ingredients" of the program or message (e.g., via costs to entry into the market or copyrights)

Behavior Change Principle-Based

- Shows target behavior.
- Shows link between behavior and (new) rewards.
- High expected present value of promised reward (temporal discounting/ uncertainty/believability of benefit).
- Causes *Surprise*: engages and attracts attention.
- Causes *Revaluation*: alters valuation of target behavior.
- Hypes the primary domain motive.
- Adds a new motive.
- Causes *Performance*: encourages target setting execution with "correct" behavior.

Communication-Based

- *Sensory*[a]: richness of channel.
- *Narrativity*: activates the imaginary mental theater that causes people to virtually experience rewards/punishments.

- *Visibility*: Makes invisible forces or causal connections visible (e.g., action of microscopic agents).
- *Sharing*: exposure causes people to go through experiences communally, so they experience social reinforcement.
- *Problematizes existing behavior*: discovers and makes evident a cost or negative consequence of existing practice (e.g., not practiced in some desirable group).

Scoring: Single point for each positive response; higher scores are better.

[a]Variable measured on dimension of low/high (with low getting the point).

---

target behavior occurs) is yet a third behavior setting: shopping at the grocery store for some new foodstuff. I assume that campaign components that require target individuals to both interpret an imaginary setting (the one in the communication) and to hold an intention to change their behavior for a long time before being able to engage in that behavior (i.e., while waiting to go to the grocery store) will be weak relative to one that has roughly the same Theory of Change mechanisms but doesn't require so much imagination or holding an intention for such a long period. Further, intervention components that require target individuals to imagine themselves playing new roles, to purchase expensive items to modify their own Target Settings, or to significantly alter their everyday routines will be less effective at changing behavior than ones that don't require such extravagancies.

The brand-based criteria in the Component Analysis Tool (Box 7.3) are familiar from marketing. Brands are important to distinguish campaigns or programs from similar ones in the marketplace; brands give program activities a coherent personality and add trust and associated values that make them cumulatively more powerful.

The behavior change principles reflect *best practice* in behavioral science terms. They are all criteria for increasing the likelihood that reinforcement learning takes place, via Surprise, Revaluation, and Performance.

Finally, the communication-based criteria largely reflect particular principles that arise from evolved aspects of human communication. For example, the ability to interpret narratives or stories via theory of mind [251] enables more complex messages to be easily digested. Ensuring that exposure to target materials takes place in a social arena is a particular means of adding force to just about any behavior. Making it explicitly clear that existing practices have some previously unnoticed negative consequence is also a powerful way of making the target behavior more likely to be selected.

FIELD TESTING

Once some initial agreement about a direction forward has been achieved, some of the central components can be tested experimentally in the field by the Creative Team (Step 3).

Concepts should be pretested prior to roll-out where possible, with additional reverts to account for any learnings in terms of interpretability, acceptability, how engaging and surprising the idea is, likeability, etc. Once everyone is satisfied with the concept and material prototypes, then the next step of development—production of intervention materials—can be performed (Step 4). See Boxes 7.4–7.6 for examples from SuperAmma design concept testing, resulting film, and other interventions, respectively.

The final job of the Creative Team is to write a report for the Deliver Team, in the form of an Implementation Manual that outlines the procedures for all intervention activities, including a time-line and logistics.

This concludes our discussion of the developmental phase of the BCD process. These first three steps—ABC—can be summarized nicely using a diagram from the field of design, the so-called double diamond (Figure 7.1) [252]. Each step can be represented by one or two diamonds, which depict the expansion and

---

Box 7.4

BCD Example

SuperAmma Concept Testing

The Creative Team rapidly identified the figure of "SuperAmma" (supermom) as the personification of the campaign ideal. As this personification was the central brand component, it was thoroughly tested in the field. Initial beliefs about the most acceptable aesthetic for the SuperAmma character (shown in the top right corner of the following illustration) proved not to be best liked. The bottom right was seen as too childish/cartoonish, while the top left was not sufficiently aspirational. The bottom left struck the most appropriate balance between being realistic yet aspirational.

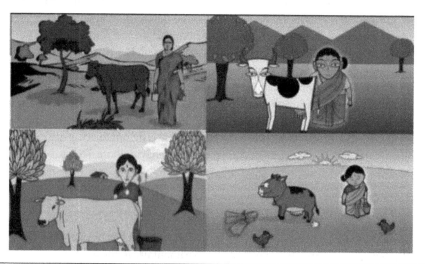

Box 7.5

BCD Example

SuperAmma Film

The essential insight, that handwashing is good manners and a characteristic of an aspirational way of life, was clearly evident in the animated film that was especially commissioned from an Indian media company, Centre of Gravity. In the film, SuperAmma's son learns to become well-mannered in many ways (including staying neat for school and respecting elders) and, as a result, goes to the city to be educated, winding up as a doctor. (This film is available at http://www.superamma.org/download-English.html.) These are powerful rewards for a diligent mother, and the grown-up son respects his mother for what she did for him when he was young as well. The narrative was achieved through multiple iterations to achieve maximum potential impact on behavior, ensuring the strongest kinds of rewards for instilling handwashing behavior (teaching handwashing is an important part of the role of being a good mother but is rewarded by improvements in the offspring's life chances and an appreciative, loving relationship with the mother), and providing the best possible role model for mothers in the target audience.

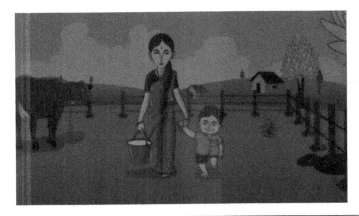

then contraction in questions or information or concepts or materials—whatever currency is relevant at that point in the development process. What the diagram makes clear is that there is a Darwinian process of generating variation in this currency and then selection of the best-fit options, resulting in a product (such as a report or plan) that gets used as the foundation for the next step. (The three central characteristics of a Darwinian process are variation, selection, and inheritance [253].) This happens over and over through each step during development. (Remember that learning can itself be seen as a Darwinian process [254].) There is thus a common dynamic running through each step, even though the currency under investigation changes from psychological ideas to physical realities along

Box 7.6

BCD EXAMPLE

SuperAmma Intervention Materials

Elements of the campaign were identified and agreed:

- Use of the SuperAmma character to personify the campaign
- An animated film to embody the central insights
- A jingle with campaign messages embedded in it
- A skit for schools
- A pledge for willing participants
- A report card for school kids to log their handwashing behavior
- The "Wall of All": a large board in the middle of the village with names of all who have pledged to wash their hands
- Posters with faces of village authorities supporting the campaign

Development of the materials and hiring of the Deliver Team was coordinated by the Creative Team in the SuperAmma case.

the way. Knowing this might help keep the process on track, as it should be obvious about what needs to happen at each point to stick to this progression.

What follows is the executional phase of Delivering the intervention and Evaluating it, which are discussed next.

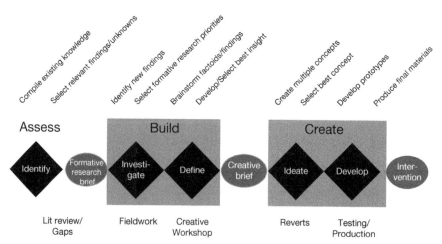

Figure 7.1. The program development process.

8

Deliver

With the intervention now designed, it can be executed. Delivery is about implementation of the intervention. Implementation is the result of program-related activities in a particular context. The Deliver Team can involve an agency specialized in conducting community events in particular kinds of circumstances (e.g., rural areas of a developing country) or a media company that arranges and supervises broadcasting schedules, for example, to facilitate delivery.

When considering alternative approaches for using channels and touchpoints, financial considerations are often paramount, and timelines can be critical. Small-scale piloting of delivery pipelines and processes are a good idea to ensure that delivery goes to plan and stays within budget.

DELIVERY STRATEGIES

Beyond providing for direct contact with the target audiences, programs can take advantage of a number of techniques for ensuring larger impacts:

- Add more role players.
  - Aim to influence the target population, both directly and indirectly, via secondary targets such as friends and neighbors or the health system.
  - Create advocates that independently begin to assist in the achievement of program objectives (e.g., by creating buzz around the program ideas that snowball through a population without further activity by the program itself).
  - Create formal partnerships with other organizations that add their authority and own activities to the program.
  - Support community action to demand change.
- Use institutions.
  - Create new groups to which target population members can belong (e.g., fan club or interest group; this can support behavior by making it a group norm or a badge of status within the group).

- Set up new training courses, change curricula, train trainers, develop institutional rules and norms, create enduring role models, set up monitoring and feedback systems, and enforce rules and laws.
- Piggyback on existing social structures to efficiently implement program activities.
- Create new institutions (e.g., via policy or production of new organization, such as a small business) that implement part of the overall plan.
- Tailor the intervention.
  - New communication technologies make it possible nowadays to modify messaging to match the state or particular characteristics of the individual receiving the communication [255].
  - Some technologies can even track changes in these characteristics over time to ensure that the most appropriate version of a message is delivered to a given individual, even as their status changes (so-called just-in-time adaptive interventions) [256].

One thing that these strategies can produce is increased layering of program activities by involving groups at various levels of organization in a nested fashion that creates strata of authority and regulation over program activities. This increases the likelihood of high-fidelity delivery. Supervision at multiple levels can reduce the likelihood of agents at any particular level deviating (for whatever reason) from program objectives. See Box 8.1 for an overview of SuperAmma delivery.

MONITORING

Monitoring is as essential to the management of behavior change programs as it is to any intervention program. Indeed, it is perhaps more so, as experience shows that surprising, innovative approaches are often resisted or perverted by actors who are more comfortable with the status quo and may have prior allegiance to other approaches. Behavior change program activities based, for example, on emotional demonstrations about disgust, can easily be turned into health education harangues by health workers, however well they have been trained, leading to a lack of fidelity to the original intention. Program managers need a comprehensive monitoring plan to track the delivery, reach, fidelity, dose, and audience response to intervention components along the Theory of Change. This requires reporting mechanisms and regular supervision and can be aided by the design of incentives paid to program actors or institutions in return for producing real, audited results—a strategy that is increasingly being used by program funding agencies.

In a perfect world, managers act on this intelligence, revising and improving the program as necessary, either on the fly or at a specified interval, for example, after a mid-term review. Sometimes feedback from sales or product uptake, for example, can be used in real time to tweak promotional messages. This will become

Box 8.1

BCD Example

SuperAmma Delivery

The SuperAmma campaign was delivered one village at a time by a pair of promoters moving around in a van that carried the materials. Two days were spent in each village.

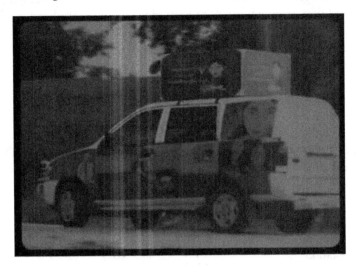

The rural activation agency delivered a campaign composed of a variety of events and interactions. For example, the largest such event involved inviting the entire community at an evening gathering during which the SuperAmma film and films of local leaders endorsing handwashing were shown, skits were played out (see photo), and community members pledged to wash their hands with soap.

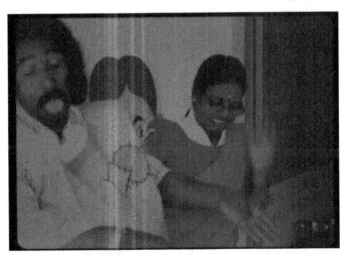

much more possible in future as large-scale programs increasingly involve electronic devices, mobile phones, smart products, or Web interactions. It is even possible in some cases to conduct small-scale experiments to see whether alternative methods of delivery might work better. However, such in-stream changes require sophisticated research designs, as well as resources that are beyond the scope of many programs at present.

It should also be recognized that there can be costs associated with flexible or adaptive programming. In industry it is common to design an intervention, set out its nonnegotiables, and then roll it out across multiple geographies. While some modifications can be made to parts of the program, the heart of it is locked down. This is to ensure the maintenance of quality, clarity, and motivation for program staff and to simplify management tasks. Endless revisions can sap energy and dilute the single-minded focus that an intervention has striven to achieve, as well as incur significant transaction costs in terms of management time, human capacity, and program resources.

Methods used for program monitoring can, and should, be both quantitative and qualitative. They should follow the Theory of Change, ensuring that the intervention is delivered, that it has modified the environment of the target audiences, that this has produced some or all of the desired changes in the

---

Box 8.2

BCD EXAMPLE

SuperAmma Delivery Problems

Implementation Issues
- The generator, sound system, or laptop on which the animated films were screened malfunctioned in some cases.
- Printers were often not available locally to print posters with faces of local people.
- School closures due to holidays, weather, or teachers' meetings inhibited performance of skits.
- The school report cards proved unsuitable for the youngest students, who were not able to follow the instructions.
- It was difficult in some cases to find or get permission to use a place for the "Wall of All."

Fidelity Issues

- Promoters learned as they went from village to village, getting better at performing the skits and ensuring there were no technological problems.

---

brains of the target audience, and that this is indeed leading to changes in behavior. If problems are diagnosed upstream (e.g., program funds have not been released to the implementer), then there is little point in looking for impacts downstream.

In large-scale behavior change programs, specialist agencies can be hired to carry out the monitoring function—for example, media monitoring specialists check that television and radio commercials have been aired as planned, that state auditors visit remote rural communities to check that local activities have taken place, and that slots can be bought in national product use surveys to examine product-purchasing behavior. Ensuring that household- or community-level activities have occurred is more daunting and expensive, as it requires field-based teams of monitors to check up on implementers in situ and in real time. (There are some means of automating this, such as requiring that implementers send in timed/dated photos of themselves engaging in expected activities prior to payment, but these checks can sometimes be gotten around as well.)

After implementation has been completed and all monitoring data have been collected, the Deliver Team should write a report or brief about the implementation problems experienced so that the Evaluation Team can have a better foundation for their process evaluation. (This can also be thought of as an implementation evaluation [257].) This can include reports from the implementing agents themselves (e.g., in the form of event logs or posthumous reflections on what went well and what didn't). An outline of SuperAmma delivery problems is provided in Box 8.2.

9

Evaluate

Finally, execution of the program should be analyzed by the Evaluation Team to learn from the experience. Traditionally, practitioners divide this task in two: first, showing that an impact has occurred as a consequence of the program (the impact evaluation) and, second, a demonstration that the hypothesized pathways of causal influence in the Theory of Change were actually achieved by the program (the process evaluation) [258–261]. The primary task of the Evaluation Team is thus to write reports concerning both the Impact and Process Evaluations.

IMPACT EVALUATION

Obviously, program managers will be anxious to know whether the program objectives have been achieved. Often, this is the only question answered by an evaluation (e.g., in a randomized controlled trial [RCT]). However, it is not always clear that the program can be held solely responsible for any observed change in the impact variables—one reason for conducting a process evaluation as well. In addition, the question of whether unintended consequences have also occurred should be addressed.

The question of how an intervention should be evaluated is a complex and contested one [262–265]. In a perfect world, a candidate behavior change intervention would be tested in a RCT against the counterfactual (the standard model) or doing nothing, depending on the investment decision to be made. Behavioral and state-of-the-world variables should be measured, program costs should be modeled, and the data should tell us whether the candidate intervention is likely to be good value for money when compared to other uses of similar investment. The RCT is the gold standard for program design, because it can make definitive statements about effects, and many scientists argue that other methods have so many methodological flaws that they are (sometimes worse than) useless [266–268].

However, RCTs are complex, expensive, and subject to a number of critiques. First, measuring a long-term outcome such as a change in mortality rates or community cohesion is likely to be prohibitively expensive in terms of sample size and, hence, resources. Second, typically only one version of the intervention can be tested, making the trial a very blunt instrument. One learns only if that particular intervention in that place and time had the desired effect. Third, while one may endeavor to deliver an intervention that can be scaled up, it is almost inevitable that in real-world conditions, some of the effect that may be seen in a trial may be diluted or lost because large-scale programs receive less intensive support and scrutiny. Fourth, there are many issues associated with the unbiased measurement of outcomes in trials, which may cast doubt on trial results. For example, previous studies with apparently excellent results in improving handwashing were possibly affected by courtesy bias; that is, participants display improved behavior differentially depending on whether they realize that the evaluation is connected with the earlier intervention [269]. There are many other types of evaluation design, some very sophisticated (e.g., propensity score matching [270]), which I do not go into here. Suffice to say that scientific impact evaluation is a specialist task that cannot be undertaken lightly.

However, behavior change interventions are also hard to evaluate because often there is no perfect, or validated, measure of behavior, so that indirect indicators have to be found. Sometimes there is a biological marker of having engaged in the target behavior, which is difficult to fake and therefore a high-quality indicator. For example, in nutritional programs, one might be able to detect the increased presence of particular micronutrients in the body of those eating recommended types of foods in their diet. But in most cases the gold standard is to actually watch what people do in the target setting after exposure to components of the intervention. This is, of course, costly and time-consuming and introduces its own biases into what is being observed (especially if the target behavior is socially desirable or normative). Self-report of changed behavior is typically the cheapest and easiest indicator and so is often used, but it is notoriously low in validity.

Despite all of these problems, it is vital that new and innovative efforts to change behavior be subject to trial, because that is how, over the years, a body of knowledge about what works to change behavior will be built up. For example, the SuperAmma trial (the results of which are shown in Box 9.1) was a complex and expensive scientific undertaking, but it represented an important step because it suggested that new approaches to behavior change for handwashing with soap—involving behavior change techniques other than health education—could be a successful way forward for public health.

Of course, it is desirable that any change achieved is sustained by the target population over the long term, although this is seldom ascertained directly by checking quantitatively at population level (at least in public health programming, where funders typically don't allocate resources for this). As a consequence, it remains difficult to provide solid, evidence-based advice about sustainability. A recent review of behavior change theory suggests that receiving continuing rewards from performance, habit formation, strong self-regulation, and social and physical environmental supports can all be important at the behavioral level [271], but evidence about what works programmatically remains lacking. It is probably an issue that depends heavily on the type of behavior being changed, aspects of

Box 9.1

BCD Example

SuperAmma Impact Evaluation

As SuperAmma is a behavior change intervention, with a ceiling of accountability stopping at behavioral outcomes, desired health impacts will be assumed to have resulted if relevant behavior change has occurred.

A small cadre of field workers did standardized observations of handwashing activity by family members in treatment and control households, first at six weeks following the intervention, with a second follow-up at 6 months and a third at 12 months. The following figure (modified from [168, Figure 3]), indicates that the target behaviors increased significantly in the intervention villages from a nearly nonexistent baseline, and these improvements were largely maintained for a year afterwards. A similar pattern was seen in the control villages when they experienced the intervention six months after the first set of villages. This is an excellent result for the first randomly clustered trial of a handwashing intervention in a developing country.

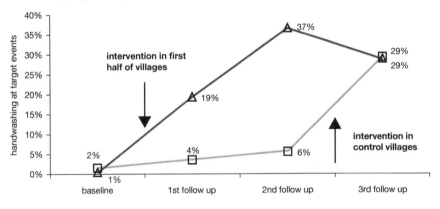

Figure source: HWWS before and after intervention, by study group. From Biran, A., et al., 2014, Effect of a behavior-change intervention on handwashing with soap in India (SuperAmma): A cluster-randomised trial. *The Lancet Global Health*, 2(3), e145–e154, licensed under CC-BY 3.0.

program deployment, and other contextual factors, so that a simple answer will not be in the offing.

Scaling up programs that have been piloted at small scale (as in the SuperAmma case) is also a major issue in program design and evaluation. Again, advice remains fairly commonsensical at this point: conduct strong management and monitoring during implementation, tailor the program to local conditions, do prior research, actively engage the range of stakeholders, provide incentives and accountability, and ensure adequate financing [272, 273]. More theoretically assured guidance on this issue awaits greater evidence but, again, may not be straightforward, as scaling up is also likely to be dependent on a number of factors.

PROCESS EVALUATION

A process evaluation is designed to understand what aspects or components of an intervention have produced the outcomes uncovered by the Outcome Evaluation. Whether the results of that evaluation are positive or poor, the process evaluation should be able to explain why. Process evaluation is built on the back of a good ongoing monitoring system during the Deliver step, and it asks similar questions, again following the logic of the Theory of Change. A good process evaluation should be able to identify several different kinds of failures that can influence program success:

- *Production problems* that delay the availability of primary materials (e.g., TV ads can take longer to create, arrange, and produce than expected leading to delays in the start date of a campaign) or make them unavailable at all (e.g., it proves impossible to find a product required for delivery of a component).
- *Logistical difficulties* in getting all the relevant players into place (e.g., subcontracting of implementation partners can run into difficulties, as when personnel wind up being unqualified or difficult to recruit or public transportation between event sites takes longer than expected).
- *Financial hitches* can escalate costs above expected levels, or market conditions like a change in exchange rates can reduce the resources available to program managers, potentially leading to a need to cut back on aspects of program delivery.
- *Contextual snags* such as holidays, national disasters, or unseasonal weather can result in an inability to deliver intervention components.
- *Faults in the Theory of Change* can occur. For example, maybe people don't actually go to the place/time selected as a touchpoint during program design (e.g., women don't buy food from the kinds of markets selected), perhaps target individuals are reluctant to participate in certain kinds of activities (e.g., don't like to engage in public commitment ceremonies), or perhaps a channel is ineffective (e.g., too much noise at the site to hear the messages being broadcast or the visual transmission was not bright enough to be seen).

These complications can result in unexpected constraints on the standard measures of process evaluation:

- *Reach* (the proportion of the target population that came into contact at least once with a component of the intervention).
- *Dose* (the number of times an average member of the target population came into contact with a given component).
- *Fidelity* (the degree to which the actual mode and tone of delivery of a component was consistent with the intended mode and tone).
- *Acceptability* (the degree to which contacts with program components were felt by target population members to not be offensive or objectionable).

The process evaluation should also be able to detect unintended consequences of the intervention. For example, promotion of some foods might actually reduce overall nutritional status due to secondary effects on cooking practices, or the food.

If a significant change in behavior *has* resulted, then the next question is usually, how can we do this better and more cheaply? Again, the process evaluation should be able to tell a plausible story about the aspects of the Theory of Change that flowed well to produce an impact and those that can be dispensed with, reducing the overall cost.

Because interventions using Behavior Centered Design (BCD) are based on an explicit theory of settings, it becomes much more likely that the learnings from one program can be abstracted and applied to another. This is because the original and new settings can be compared with the likelihood of applicability being a function of how similar the two settings are. A good BCD process evaluation can, therefore, "pan for gold," seeking to pick out the "active ingredients" of an intervention, which will be replicable in other circumstances.

The BCD tool for conducting a process evaluation (outlined in Box 9.2) refers again to the elements of the Theory of Change. Each aspect should be measured as best as possible with available resources. For example, in the SuperAmma process evaluation, we documented all of the inputs, tried to trace the impact that the intervention had had on the environment (e.g., that in some villages there was no place to put our public display of commitment by village members), and asked a simple set of formal questions to a population sample concerning psychological responses to the intervention (see Box 9.3).

The SuperAmma process evaluation indicated that there had been widespread exposure to the campaign, that it had affected relevant beliefs, as well as behavior (as seen in the impact evaluation; see Box 9.1). These psychological changes were in line with expectations from the campaign's Theory of Change, which lends credibility to the results.

Finally, cost-effectiveness is another consideration, especially if one is thinking of scaling up a program or attempting to convince others to adapt it for their own uses. The SuperAmma trial was investigated (in terms of delivery, not overall

Box 9.2

BCD Tool

Process Evaluation Components List

- Implementation (environmental changes)
  - Context within which implementation took place
    - Sociopolitical/economic conditions
    - Other projects/programs
  - Exposure to project-specific elements (with frequency/dosage)
  - Proportion of target population reached with each type of exposure (reach)
  - Fidelity of implementation to intervention plan (management of delivery)
    - Touchpoint-based failures
    - Activity-based failures
    - Channel-based failures
    - Behavior Change Technique-based failures
- Outputs (psychological changes)
  - Plans/beliefs (including norms)
  - Motive salience
  - Automaticity of performance
- Outcomes (behavioral changes)
  - Target behavior frequency
  - Contextual determinants of performance
- Impacts (state-of-the-world changes)
  - New psychological/performance abilities
  - Psychological well-being
  - Institutions/organizations (i.e., ways of social working)
- Physical infrastructures (e.g., sidewalks)

development; see Box 9.4), which put the cost of the intervention at about $2,000 per village, which compares favorably with other public health investments, suggesting that it could be a candidate for replication [274].

DISSEMINATION

The last actions the Program Team need to conduct are to agree on the content of the evaluation reports and on the next phase of activities (e.g., a repeat of the process, or scaling up of the existing program, potentially modified in some ways from what has been learned). Evaluation results are important, not just to inform the next

Box 9.3

BCD Example

SuperAmma Process Evaluation

A variety of measures were taken as indicators confirming the existence, and use of, the causal pathways predicted by the Theory of Change for this program:

- Exposure was confirmed by questions concerning informant knowledge of campaign-specific information, such as the campaign brand elements (the ability to recognize the figure of SuperAmma, the campaign jingle, etc.).
- Reported attendance at campaign events.
- Changes in variables concerning the value of the target behaviors in control and intervention villages were compared between intervention and control villages.

Analysis of the responses suggested that there had been a substantial revaluation of handwashing in campaign villages: handwashing was more often seen as being good manners and was more often seen as "what everyone does round here," suggesting that norms around handwashing had changed significantly. Handwashing also became seen as a nurturing act and one that might enhance social status. We therefore concluded that elements of our approach were responsible for the success of the campaign, although we don't know which elements had the biggest impact.

Response	Intervention (%)	Control (%)
HWWS is good manners.	84	21
HWWS protects children.	63	2
HWWS leads to success in life.	30	0
Everybody around here washes their hands with soap.	35	8

HWWS = handwashing with soap.

program cycle, but also for other behavior change practitioners. Hence, publication in a publicly available form, ideally after peer review, is important. The impact and process evaluations can be written up for internal consumption only (i.e., as project reports) or disseminated more broadly (e.g., as academic papers) and constitute the ultimate learnings from having conducted the program. (In the case of the SuperAmma project, both reports were published as academic papers [168, 274].)

Box 9.4

BCD Example

SuperAmma Cost-Effectiveness

In this case, cost-effectiveness was measured very simply, essentially to provide an estimate of the cost of scaling up for interested nongovernment and governmental organizations.

Item	Cost (USD)
Equipment	
Purchased	2,425
Hired	4,378
Intervention materials	
Nonconsumables	356
Human resources	3,915
Staff Hire	4978
Total Cost	16,053
Cost Per Village	2,293

If results are positive and if the new program designed using BCD is good value for money, then it is vital also that policymakers learn about it and learn from it. In the case of SuperAmma, the creative agency built a dedicated website to lodge all of the materials, made a short animation explaining how the intervention worked and the results, and efforts were made to pass the results to the Indian Government in various forms (ongoing). A major soap producer is now scaling up the intervention, and it is being adapted to various countries in Africa and Asia.

Conducting a full circuit of BCD (i.e., all five alphabetic steps) as I have described here should ideally be seen as simply one iteration of a longer-term process. Populations have a history, and this often means they have been exposed to multiple behavior change programs, often with respect to the same behaviors, prior to the present campaign, and will be again afterwards. Trust can be crucial to the success of both today's as well as tomorrow's campaign. Indeed, a large part of the value of a campaign can be due to development of this trust, the result of relationships formed over time through repeated interaction between consumers and companies, or government agencies and the general public.

We can, therefore, think of an implicit sixth step in the process, the F step—call it *follow-up*—to ensure that lessons are learned and incorporated into any future programming. This would close the circle of learning as it feeds back into itself via the A step (Assess) of the next project.

10

What's Next?

I'll end this presentation of the Behavior Centered Design (BCD) approach with a few comments on how the approach can be extended to other kinds of behavior change projects and what might hold for its future. I then conclude with a few reflections on how we can all learn how to "do behavior change" better.

EXTENSIONS

In this book, presentation of the BCD approach and process has been couched in terms of developing a standard communication- or activity-based campaign (e.g., for public health or marketing purposes). However, much the same approach and process can be employed with respect to other kinds of behavior change projects. Here, I'll discuss these alternative uses briefly through illustrative (simplified) scenarios.

Policy-Based Change

In the case of seeking to change public policy, the immediate target of behavior change is not a fairly general demographic (as was true of public health programs) but rather a specific and relatively small class of people, or perhaps even a single individual—that is, one or more policymakers. Use of the BCD approach in this case forces recognition that policymakers are individuals who need motivation, who play specific roles in particular settings and perform particular behaviors (like signing policy into law), just like anyone else. Take the following scenario as an example.

A former US senator starts a political lobbying group in Washington, DC, called Smoke-Free, with the mission to promote federal antismoking legislation (outcome), so that rates of lung cancer in the United States can be reduced by inhibiting the number of people taking up this practice (impact).

Assess: The lobbying organization's staffers write a background document (White Paper) on the scientific evidence for a link between smoking and lung cancer, as well as a document on the means by which other lobbying groups successfully gained access to policy-makers or caused changes in public opinion (e.g., through publicity-seeking).

Build: The staff develop a BCD Theory of Change to direct their efforts at convincing lawmakers of the need for a new policy (e.g., by causing them to cause the policymaker to revalue the value of the target behavior for his constituents and writing up a draft proposal of the relevant policy to ease the job for legislators) and a separate Theory of Change about their efforts to change public opinion (where the target population is again a general demographic).

Create: Smoke-Free goes to a professional media company to help them with tag lines, poster design, and radio ads (all they can afford) as materials to be used in their publicity campaign; staffers themselves write the draft legislation to make it easy for interested policymakers.

Deliver: Smoke-Free targets legislators directly by meeting with the staff of crucial legislators, passing on their evidence base and use motivational patter to persuade these seconds-in-command about the justice of their cause. Simultaneously, they target the general public via media campaigns to change public opinion so that this secondary target demographic takes up behaviors that will support their cause and apply pressure on the lawmakers. These include attending constituent meetings of the legislators likely to vote against such a proposition. The result is that the sought-for policy fails to be written into law.

Evaluate: The lobbying group performs an internal assessment of its strategy (i.e., process evaluation) to identify the reasons it failed to have the desired impact and develops plans for a second attempt during the next political cycle using a revised Theory of Change.

Business Development

Ms. Smith makes a business pitch to Ms. Jones, a serial entrepreneur and venture capitalist, concerning her idea for a new kind of mousetrap that will markedly improve its ability to catch mice. Ms. Jones decides to take the case on, to see if the device can serve as the primary product of a new, profitable manufacturing and retail company (impact).

Assess: Ms. Jones engages in some research into the market for the improved product and determines the idea is worth further investigation.

Build: Ms. Jones then develops two different Theories of Change: one to check if there is a way to produce the potential product at a profit via a business that relies primarily on production and sale of this product, using the BCD Theory of Change to help organize her thoughts about how the product can be engineered and then sold to consumers with a particular profile. She also uses the BCD Theory of Change to guide her efforts to get financial backing for a new business (which involves crowd-sourcing and personal contacts to get an initial round of funding for the small business that will produce and market the device).

Create: Using the crowd-sourced money, Ms. Jones hires an engineering firm to create prototypes of the new product, which are iteratively refined over a couple of years through repeated consumer piloting and redesign using the BCD Component Analysis Tool. Simultaneously, she hires a creative agency to design a marketing campaign for the product, whose reverts are critiqued using the BCD Component Analysis Tool. Third, she also hires a variety of personnel to form the foundation of the small business that will eventually manage production, distribution, marketing, sales and servicing of the new product.

Deliver: The new company, Acme Ltd., begins production, achieves a stockpile of merchandise, is publicly launched via news announcements to the business press, and initiates the marketing plan. Sales begin to come in, which are tracked.

Evaluate: After the first year of business, Ms. Jones has some of her staff write a market report (for internal consumption only) to look at company profitability (i.e., the impact evaluation) and the level of customer satisfaction with the product and the viability of their servicing model (i.e., process evaluation).

Marketing

Sales of a new kind of mousetrap are not increasing as fast as the Acme Ltd. company believes is possible, despite several different marketing efforts. They desire to increase both the market share and the market size for this product (outcomes), as a means to greater company profits (impact).

Assess: Acme hires an external research agency, Beta Research, to prepare a background report on market conditions and sales over the time of the prior marketing pushes.

Build: Beta Research also conducts some consumer research to uncover reasons for the lack of appeal of prior marketing campaigns to target consumers (using the BCD Campaign Analysis Tool to help design the research). In a meeting between Acme and Beta staff, consensus is reached about a new Theory of Change for targeting the brand profile of consumer and a creative brief for the new marketing campaign is written.

Create: The Acme company uses their regular creative agency, Create-Great, to design storyboards for a new TV and radio ad. These are critiqued through several iterations using the BCD Component Analysis Tool

before being accepted by Acme management and then produced by a
media production company subcontracted by Create-Great.

Deliver: Create-Great then follows an implementation plan previously
created by Acme together with Beta Research to broadcast the ads in
particular markets at particular times of day to maximize reach and the
dosage of exposure, given their budget.

Evaluate: Acme management commissions an internal report to examine
whether objectives were met (i.e., the impact evaluation), with particular
attention to the cost-effectiveness of the different kinds of broadcasts, to
improve financial efficiency over the next advertising cycle (i.e., process
evaluation).

Self-Help

Mr. Brown wakes up one morning in a hotel room he doesn't recognize and
realizes he is isn't sure which city he is in or what day it is. He immediately vows to
reduce his consumption of alcohol, so as to enjoy a better quality of life.

Assess: Having made this commitment to himself, Mr. Brown buys a couple
of self-help books for alcoholics and reads them.

Build: Having learned in the books about Alcoholics Anonymous (AA) and
their excellent record of getting alcoholics to quit drinking, he searches
for local AA meetings on the Web, and finds one that conveniently meets
nearby his workplace on Wednesday nights. (AA has a very explicit
Theory of Change for how to convert alcoholics into nondrinkers,
relying heavily upon recovering alcoholics as therapists, peer-led self-
help therapy groups, and teaching the 12-step process, including self-
identification as an alcoholic, which Mr. Brown—at least implicitly—has
found compelling during his reading.)

Create: Mr. Brown consciously produces a plan for how to incorporate
AA meetings into his life. He clears his calendar of other activities on
AA meeting nights and plans how to get to the meeting place on time
from work.

Deliver: He goes to his first AA meeting the following Wednesday. He finds
the experience so rewarding that he goes again the next week, and the
next. He finds that he is learning techniques that will help him to quit.
Together with others in the AA group, he plans his quit date. When it
comes, he quits drinking outright.

Evaluate: After three months of sobriety, Mr. Brown is asked in one of
the AA meetings to reflect on his experience (i.e., conduct a process
evaluation) and share it with others in the group (to have further impact
on himself, and others, via the AA Theory of Change).

This suite of scenarios should help demonstrate that the BCD approach is quite general to any organizational process that involves changing behavior in any population (down to a single individual).

FUTURE DEVELOPMENTS

A number of capabilities are coming online that can be built into the BCD process, mostly based on technological advances related to behavioral science. The first advance, which we are beginning to make use of, is agent-based modeling. This is an analytical technique that was developed to understand complex systems in a range of physical, biological, and social sciences. It arose from a need to understand the behavior that emerges from the many interactions between different individual elements within a system. For example, it is being used to understand the flocking behavior of birds, the spread of diseases through a population, and the causes of boom and bust in housing markets.

These simulations act as market laboratories that provide organizations a source of insight about behavior and the power to experiment with potential strategies to address questions such as

- Why do people behave in the way that is observed?
- What are the most important influences on behavior?
- What might happen in the future in a range of scenarios?
- What data should be collected to improve our understanding?

The technique is particularly applicable to analyze and understand populations where

- There are many interdependent influences on behavior.
- It is hard to run experiments in the real world.
- There are multifarious types of social interactions.

While agent-based modeling has been around for over 30 years, a wider set of enabling techniques has only emerged recently to allow the development of robust, large-scale simulations of human behavior, including

- Insights from behavioral psychology that allow the development of stronger rules of individual behavior.
- The availability of a wider range of data that can be used to validate simulations.
- Cloud computing that provides low cost, scalable computing resources which can be used to run large volumes of simulations cost effectively.

- Big data analysis techniques that can deal with the large volumes of data generated by simulations.
- Common software platforms such as NetLogo and AnyLogic.

These developments, taken together, bring more powerful agent-based modeling within the capabilities of more people.

I believe that agent-based modeling can be used throughout the BCD process to help develop and test the causal claims in a program's Theory of Change. It can be coupled with statistical analysis of evaluation-based data to confirm particular links.

A second major future development concerns behavior *monitoring*. Existing methods for observing behavior have been subject to a fundamental problem: people, like subatomic particles, react to being observed. In effect, the act of looking itself influences what is seen (an analogue of the Heisenberg Uncertainty Principle). People change what they are doing if they know they are being watched and don't tell the truth when reporting on their own behavior (e.g., to avoid embarrassing or idiosyncratic activities). An ideal solution would be a system that can tell what people are doing without itself being obtrusive.

Many researchers have been developing smart home systems to monitor everyday activities in a way that largely avoids Heisenberg's paradox. However, these systems are ad hoc, composed of multiple kinds of devices (e.g., RFID tags, cameras, microphones, infrared presence detectors, temperature/humidity sensors), complex, and fragile and hence difficult to install or maintain. They often provide a level of detail (e.g., about body orientation) that is not necessary for activity recognition.

On the other hand, there are a number of commercially available, relatively simple and robust systems for monitoring activity in home environments. For example, Care Innovation's QuietCare, and Just Checking systems both consist of wireless passive infrared units, together with a base unit that plugs into the wall mains for power, and report periodically to a website. They can be left in place for months at a time, are unobtrusive, relatively easy to install, and cost-effective. However, they are restricted to detecting gross levels of activity (usually by a single person) in given rooms of the house. In effect, they enable macro-scale routine estimation (e.g., time spent in bathroom), not monitoring of behavioral sequences within such spaces—that is, they don't actually get at daily routines and so can't really inform behavior change efforts.

For the past several years, I have been developing (with colleagues) a new kind of smart home system that falls between these two extremes, enabling the robust detection of specific behaviors in natural environments. We have adapted a real-time location system (RTLS), normally designed for industrial or institutional use, for use in households [275]. RTLS has a number of desirable characteristics:

- *Integrated*: single components manufacturer, on a single electrical bus.
- *Robust*: shock- and water-proof commercial-grade components (used in industrial contexts such as hospitals and warehouses), with redundant

communication protocols, mean the system can be left undisturbed for months at a time.

- *Simple*: uses only four kinds of components—person/object Tags, Exciters to define specific detection zones, a Reader for managing the Exciters and Tags, and a plug computer for storing/transmitting data to the Web.
- *Flexible*: with a range of sensitivities to inputs, configurations of components, novel types of components, components able to communicate across significant distances.
- *Scalable*: additional behaviors can be studied simply by adding tags to the relevant objects.
- *Unobtrusive*: components are small in size and blend into the background, with limited wiring.
- *Accurate*: low rates of data loss ensure few false negatives; false positives can be managed through use of contextual information.
- *Cost-effective*: around $1,300 per system, which can be used for many installations.

Use of an RTLS is justified on the basis that most behaviors of interest require people to interact with focal objects (e.g., a soap dispenser for handwashing, toothpaste, medicine bottle, kettle, oven, bed, etc.). By having people wear a watch-like sensor and tagging the objects required to perform each of the target behaviors, we can tell who is doing what and where and when they are doing it (thanks to other features of the system). Thus, the system enables us to monitor a wide range of behaviors, and because we can cost-effectively monitor many behaviors by the same people on a day-to-day basis simply by adding sensors to more objects around the house, we can measure regularity in the sequencing and timing of daily routines.

I believe use of RTLS in home and work environments holds tremendous promise for the scientific study of behavior in situ, over the long term, cost-effectively, and with minimal interference. It should become the new standard for conducting behavioral studies of all kinds.

REFLECTIONS

Three general classes of science can be distinguished, based on the degree to which they study phenomena under human control and manipulation. Observational sciences are those in which *nothing* is under control (e.g., history, sociology, natural history). Experimental sciences are those in which *everything* (relevant) is under control (e.g., physics, chemistry, and lab sciences). Intervention sciences are those in which *something* is under control (e.g., public health, political science, pharmacy).

In the observational sciences, one can look at historical patterns of change or process (e.g., rise and fall of civilizations), tease out interesting cause–effect linkages, or use cross-sectional designs to examine correlations. Typically, one just looks at variation in one time slice or at some sequence of events and postulate a causal account (e.g., history). This is generally considered weak science as correlation is not causation, and one can't be sure about the presence of confounding factors that actually should figure in any explanatory account.

In the experimental sciences, the scientist introduces a factor into a well-known situation (e.g., a second chemical into a test tube full of something), but since all the irrelevant variables can be accounted for (ideally by being held constant), any change in the outcome (e.g., a new substance) is considered to be the result of the proposed mechanism (e.g., a chemical reaction with theorized properties). A simple before/after design is typically sufficient in these sciences: does the expected change in the outcome variable occur? If so, the hypothesis is considered to be confirmed. A few replications may be required when there are multiple factors involved that might have some influence, but otherwise, testing is considered to be pretty conclusive.

In the intervention sciences the *something* that is under control is the intervention. Typically, some factor is introduced into the wild (e.g., a human population), with the hope that some desired change is produced in the chosen outcome. In such cases, the connection between the cause (intervention) and effect (outcome) can be fuzzy, as many things may change as a consequence of the intervention or due to other processes happening simultaneously, so you can't be sure that changes in the outcome variable are due to the intervention. Behavior change and program design obviously fall into the category of intervention science. This book can be seen as an attempt to introduce material from experimental science into intervention science via development of the BCD approach. In particular, evolutionary biology is *the* science of change. Reinforcement learning is *the* theory outlining the changes that happen as a consequence of behavior. These are the natural foundations of a science of behavior change; they are the foundations of the BCD approach.

The BCD approach is also able to encompass factors ranging from the psychological to the macro-sociological in one coherent conceptual framework issuing from behavioral theory. BCD clearly sets out a necessary and sufficient chain of events that must occur to generate behavior change and provides a raft of theory-based tools to help with that task.

What gives BCD its conceptual unity is its focus on *learning*, which is the way in which all change occurs, whether at individual, organizational, or program level. In fact, BCD contains a hierarchy of learning models:

- *Individual-level learning*: the BCD Behavior Change Model is a reinforcement learning model embedded in a behavior setting.
- *Organizational-level learning*: the BCD Theory of Change Model embedded in the center of the Behavior Change Process Model concerns how individuals or organizations themselves learn from exposure to an intervention.

- *Program-level learning*: the ABCDE steps in the BCD Program Process Model describe program execution as a set of processes that result in learning from the experience of developing and implementing the program itself.

The fact that the models are hierarchically embedded ensures that they are consistent with one another as well as being theoretically grounded.

The BCD process has been presented in quite linear fashion, for simplicity. However, each step can involve iterative learning—the Assess step can make a first effort at defining target behaviors but then reformulate them in the light of new information from background searches or critique by an expert. Formative research during the Build step will always begin with one set of questions but end up with another set and can include field-based experiments that test initial hypotheses about the form and/or content of the eventual intervention, to reduce the number of live options prior to handing off to the Create Team. The Create step is a process that can involve numerous generations of idea invention, plus quick, small-scale field testing, and refinement prior to roll out of the finished intervention. Delivery can also be iterative in some cases; if monitoring picks up ways that implementation is deviating from plan, this operational failure can be corrected. Similarly, if some element of the expected psychological change has not occurred (a Theory of Change failure), then new activities can be arranged. Finally, the Evaluate Team can go back to the field to try to learn what went wrong, isolate particular causal pathways, and, hence, reconsider the final lessons from program execution. The degree to which iterative testing and refinement take place at each step is a function of the time, financing, and technical capabilities available to the program. The basic rule is that it is always easier to test early and test often than to risk rolling out a campaign at scale that is not as effective as it could be.

The basic principle of BCD is, *Disrupt settings with Surprise to force Revaluation and so cause Performance*. This principle reflects the logic of the BCD Theory of Change, from the Behavior Change Challenge viewpoint, which suggests that interventions modify environments in ways that influence psychological processes in predictive brains such that new actions are chosen. The Theory of Change is central to the entire BCD process and describes how this disruption is expected to arise: the Assess and Build steps (through formative research) identify a program's Theory of Change, the Create step produces materials and the Delivery step produces a strategy that will lead to the desired outputs and impact, and documents from the Evaluate step determine whether the Theory of Change (and its hypothesized mechanisms) are a true description of what happened during implementation. I can summarize the essential behavior change requirement as one of having to *reset* some important facet of the relevant situation so that regular reinforcement learning can occur, and the target behavior becomes the natural outcome of all the forces at work.

The BCD approach divides the program development and execution process into five steps (note the mnemonic of ABCDE):

- *Assess*: determine what is known and unknown about current and desired behaviors and their determinants.
- *Build*: fill in the knowledge gaps by collecting data (e.g., through formative research).
- *Create*: produce the concepts and materials that will have an impact on the program objective.
- *Deliver*: execute the plan to expose the target population to the program's activities.
- *Evaluate*: determine whether the predicted environmental, psychological and behavioral changes occurred.

It is interesting to note that this process can itself be expressed as a form of reinforcement learning:

- Assess = recognition of a problem from some stimulus.
- Build = interpretation and contextualization of the problem/stimulus.
- Create = development of a potential response.
- Deliver = behavioral activity/response (body-environment interaction).
- Evaluate = learning from environmental feedback.

The steps identified by the BCD process thus describe an organizational learning process that is similar to the reinforcement learning happening at the individual level. Of course, any good behaviour change program should result in those associated with the program having learned important lessons that can then be applied to future programs of a similar kind. Using a BCD process makes this more likely to happen, as it is couched explicitly in processes based on learning.

Further, this learning process should be cumulative, as the organizations behind program development take learnings from each iteration of the BCD process into the development of subsequent programs. Only in this way can we all get better at achieving socially desirable impacts through behavior change programs— whether to improve public health, to modify policy, form a company to sell a new product, or help oneself to improve one's own behavior. Having a unified theoretical and practical approach for all of these kinds of problems should only increase the rate at which we all learn from such varied experiences of behavior change.

ACKNOWLEDGMENTS

For reading previous versions and intellectual inputs, many thanks go to Weston Baxter, Adam Biran, Om Prasad Gautam, Katie Greenland, Sharon Guten, Jessie deWitt Huberts, Ron Hess, Gaby Judah, Hans-Joachim Mosler, Maddie Sands, Ben Tidwell, Robert West, Sian White, Allan Wicker, and several anonymous reviewers.

Also, my gratitude goes to Balaji Gopalan from Centre of Gravity (now Upward Spiral) and Jaykrishnan Menon (now of Applied Wonder) for their inspired SuperAmma materials (and BCD logo); Randy Bakes, Helen Trevaskis, Crispen Sachikonye, and Irene Jeffries for various creative inputs; and Sarah Harrington and those at Oxford University Press who shepherded this book along.

Finally, Val Curtis played a number of important roles: co-developer of BCD, sounding board, manuscript reader, and life partner. Thanks don't cover it.

CHAPTER 1

1. The BCD RL model is not a psychological model in the sense of including extensive predictions about information processing in the brain—that is, it does not specify particular relationships between mental constructs as can be seen (e.g., in the Health Belief Model [2]) and the expectancy-value approaches such as the Theory of Planned Behavior [56]. This is because the model is couched at a higher level of abstraction, including many different kinds of causal factors than just cognitive ones. I don't believe this to be a liability, but rather a strength, as it is much more likely that the important causes of behavior will be discovered by a broader search through the kinds of factors this approach emphasizes.

2. Basic RL models make learning and memory equivalent to the act of perceiving new states of the world; here we distinguish two separate steps: perception of the consequences of behavior and the mental processes of making inferences from what is perceived (learning) and then storage of those inferences (memory). This is closer in psychological terms to what happens in brains.

3. Health psychologists have called *temporal imbalance* behaviors "health-enhancing" or "health protective," while *super-stimulating* behaviors have been termed "health-risk" or "health compromising" [72, 73], albeit without the same theoretical underpinnings as provided here.

4. People may also not take up new technologies because they do not have access to them. This can occur when people live in the ancestral state of preindustrial lifestyles where the primary causes of early death are violence and pathogens. Temporal imbalance in these cases has become a problem because the modern world has introduced new solutions, which relatively poor people are not in position to adopt.

5. A number of caveats should be noted here. Many factors can come into play before a learning problem becomes a public health problem: many people must exhibit the learning deficit, the environment must be characterized in specific way for the learning problem to arise and persist (foiling the evolutionary "tinkering" of learning mechanisms), the learning deficit must relate to a significant health outcome, a tenable solution must be evident (or the problem simply has no solution), and social institutions must recognize the problem as a problem. Also, admittedly, behavior is only one aspect of these problems: for example, the AIDS epidemic is also caused by challenges to the human immune system presented by

a fast-evolving, virulent virus, and undernutrition caused by geopolitical and eco-nomic inequalities. Further, in some cases, a public health intervention need not require behavior change at all. For example, iodine was introduced into salt in some countries by governmental decree, producing health benefits for the population, but without requiring people to engage in any novel behavior or to stop doing anything in particular, but simply to continue consuming salt. Nevertheless, we have shown there is a common link between all major global public health problems, which is that the behavioral underpinnings—such as inadequate uptake of condoms or ad-herence to antiretroviral therapy in the case of AIDS—can be explained as a kind of inappropriate or unfortunate learning and that there are strong linkages between these learning difficulties, behavioral problems, risk factors, and public health issues.

CHAPTER 2

1. For public health practitioners, it is important to recognize that hyping up health benefits is unlikely to make people experience (or imagine) any immediate, tangible reward for behavior. Indeed, health is not one of the 15 human motives; we did not evolve a reward system for healthy behavior, as such. Hence, messaging about health consequences is unlikely to be an effective strategy for public health behavior change efforts [76].

2. It is important to note that this level of organization occurs between the individual and the usual social scientific concept of an organization, such as a business or school. In particular, multiple settings can occur within the operation of a social organization (e.g., "Mrs. Smith's music class" within a school or the "weekly staff meeting" within a government bureau). This makes Barker's notion of a setting different from the setting concept used in health promotion, or the World Health Organization's "healthy setting" concept, which equate a setting with a hospital, village, or other social organization [81, 82]. When necessary, the phrase *behavior setting* will be utilized to ensure the ecological psychological notion is distinguished from this other use.

CHAPTER 3

1. This model was previously called the Evo-Eco model [95].

2. Recent evidence suggests that plants can communicate with one another chemically (as do some animals), but their behavior is highly constrained compared to most animals.

3. What happens inside a computer can also be described using Newtonian principles, although it might require quite a long description.

4. There are some liminal objects or states of being: artificially intelligent objects, capable of a strategic response, but without genes, lie between the biological and physical environments. Dead animals and people can probably be considered to form part of the physical environment, as their genes are no longer active or rele-vant, and these objects don't strategize any longer.

5. They don't, however, make manipulable objects, with the exception of a few spiders, which make webs that they can maneuver about with their legs.

6. Here, I exclude the complex dwelling creation conducted by social insects such as termites, which create large structures using a particular kind of rigid mechanism

(stigmergy) [221] or the transformation of soil layers by earthworms through continual digestion of their surroundings. These mechanisms are unlike the highly creative production process used by humans.

7. Existing theories of behavior change such as Self-Regulation theory, the ABC approach, and the Transtheoretical Model do not recognize the impact of one behavior on another. They think of behavior in abstract terms, such as stopping smoking or eating a healthy diet—behaviors that are obviously complex in many ways, including temporally.

8. This argument for evolutionary precursors to human forms of behavior settings is novel here; it is not characteristic of the Barker school in ecological psychology, where the concept of a behavior setting originated. Placing the notion of a behavior setting into this evolutionary framework makes it closer to Caporael's repeated assembly concept [195], which involves organisms, artifacts and practices being repeatedly put together for interaction as a unit of natural selection. Repeated assemblies are "recurrent entity-environment relations composed of hierarchically organized heterogeneous components having different temporal frequencies and scales of replication." Thus, although more general (genes are taken as an example), this concept should include behavior settings as an example.

9. A related notion is that of affordance, associated with Gibson [205]. However, it is not as specific, nor part of as powerful an ecology of ideas, as developed by the Barker school.

CHAPTER 4

1. We can also link the tasks associated with the BCD Behavior Change Challenge to the elements of the BCD Theory of Change (which is at the center of the BCD process diagram; see Figure 4.1). As the Theory of Change diagram shows, three causal links must be made: from Surprise to Revaluation to Performance (which result in changes to the state of the world that the program seeks to influence). Since Surprise, Revaluation, and Performance are glosses on implementation, outputs, and outcomes, this model demonstrates a tight connection between a fundamental learning process and the BCD requirements for developing a clear Theory of Change—an integration not previously achieved in the Theory of Change literature.

CHAPTER 6

1. Note, however, that branding is not always a good thing: in some cases, the desired impact can be achieved through other means. For example, a campaign to reduce injuries on railway lines in India employed markings on the track that changed the perception of the speed of the oncoming train and so stopped people thinking they could cross the tracks in time (http://finalmile.in/behaviorarchitecture/category/irrationality/safety)—a purely environmental implementation to which people respond subconsciously and which would work less well if people were made aware of the manipulation, much less have been branded. In such cases, the branding-related criteria should be ignored.

REFERENCES

1. Curtis, V., & Aunger, R. (2011). Motivational mismatch: Evolved motives as the source of—and solution to—global public health problems. In S. C. Roberts (Ed.), *Applied evolutionary psychology* (pp. 259–275). Oxford, England: Oxford University Press.
2. Becker, M., Drachman, R., & Kirscht, J. (1974). A new approach to explaining sick-role behavior in low-income populations. *American Journal of Public Health, 64,* 205–216.
3. Ajzen, I., & Fishbein, M. (1973). Attitudinal and normative variables as predictors of specific behavior. *Journal of Personality and Social Psychology, 27,* 41–57.
4. Bandura, A. (1977). Self-efficacy: Toward a unifying theory of behavioral change. *Psychological Review, 84,* 191–215.
5. Sunstein, C., & Thaler, R. (2008). *Nudge: Improving decisions about health, wealth, and happiness.* New Haven, CT: Yale University Press.
6. Ariely, D. (2009). *Predictably irrational.* New York, NY: HarperCollins.
7. Michie, S., van Stralen, M. M., & West, R. (2011). The behaviour change wheel: A new method for characterising and designing behaviour change interventions. *Implementation Science, 6,* 42.
8. Devine, J. (2009). *Introducing SaniFOAM: A framework to analyze sanitation behaviors to design effective sanitation programs.* Washington, DC: Water and Sanitation Program.
9. Batra, R., & Ray, M. L. (1986). Situational effects of advertising repetition: The moderating influence of motivation, ability, and opportunity to respond. *Journal of Consumer Research, 12,* 432–445.
10. Rothschild, M. (1999). Carrots, sticks and promises: A conceptual framework for the behaviour management of public health and social issues. *Journal of Marketing, 63,* 24–37.
11. Funder, D. C. (2009). Persons, behaviors and situations: An agenda for personality psychology in the postwar era. *Journal of Research in Personality, 43*(2), 120–126.
12. Yang, Y., Read, S. J., & Miller, L. (2009). The concept of situations. *Social and Personality Psychology Compass, 3*(6), 1018–1037.
13. Fleeson, W., & Noftle, E. E. (2009). The end of the person-situation debate: An emerging synthesis in the answer to the consistency question. *Social and Personality Psychology Compass, 2,* 1667–1684.
14. Odling-Smee, F. J., Laland, K. N., & Feldman, M. (2003). *Niche construction: The neglected process in evolution.* Princeton, NJ: Princeton University Press.
15. Friston, K. (2010). The free-energy principle: A unified brain theory? *Nature Reviews Neuroscience, 11*(2), 127–138.
16. Aunger, R., & Curtis, V. (2016). Behaviour centred design: Towards an applied science of behaviour change. *Health Psychology Review, 10*(4), 425–446.

17. Schultz, W. (2006). Behavioral theories and the neurophysiology of reward. *Annual Review of Psychology, 57,* 87–115.

18. Scott, J. (2000). Rational choice theory. In G. Browning, A. Halcli, & F. Webster (Eds.), *Understanding contemporary society: Theories of the present* (pp. 129–138). London, England: SAGE.

19. Hupp, S. D., Reitman, D., & Jewell, J. D. (2008). Cognitive-behavioral theory. In M. Hersen & A. M. Gross (Eds.), *Handbook of clinical psychology: Vol. 2. Children and adolescents.* New York, NY: Wiley.

20. Martínez-Meyer, E., Townsend Peterson, A., & Hargrove, W. W. (2004). Ecological niches as stable distributional constraints on mammal species, with implications for Pleistocene extinctions and climate change projections for biodiversity. *Global Ecology and Biogeography, 13*(4), 305–314.

21. Wyles, J., Kunkel, J., & Wilson, A. (1983). Birds, behavior, and anatomical evolution. *Proceedings of the National Academy of Sciences of the United States of America, 80,* 4394–4397.

22. Wcislo, W. (1989). Behavioral environments and evolutionary change. *Annual Review of Ecology and Systematics, 20,* 137–169.

23. Huey, R., Hertz, P., & Sinervo, B. (2003). Behavioral drive versus behavioral inertia in evolution: A null model approach. *American Naturalist, 161,* 357–366.

24. Sterelny, K. (2003). *Mind in a hostile world.* Oxford, England: Oxford University Press.

25. Freeman, W. J. (1999). *How the brain makes up its mind.* London, England: Weidenfeld and Nicholson.

26. Tinbergen, N. (1963). On aims and methods of ethology. *Zeitschrift fur Tierpsychologie, 20,* 410–433.

27. Plotkin, H. (1988). Learning and evolution. In H. Plotkin (Ed.), *The role of behavior in evolution.* Cambridge, MA: MIT Press.

28. Millikan, R. G. (2000). *On clear and confused ideas: An essay about substance concepts.* Cambridge, England: Cambridge University Press.

29. Richerson, P. J., & Boyd, R. (2005). *Not by genes alone: How culture transformed human evolution.* Chicago, IL: University of Chicago Press.

30. Quartz, S. (2001). Toward a developmental evolutionary psychology: Genes, development, and the evolution of human cognitive architecture. In S. Scher & M. Rauscher (Eds.), *Evolutionary psychology: Alternative approaches.* Boston, MA: Kluwer.

31. Potts, R. (2012). Evolution and environmental change in early human prehistory. *Annual Review of Anthropology, 41,* 151–167.

32. Sutton, R. S. (1984). *Temporal credit assignment in reinforcement learning* (Doctoral dissertation). University of Massachusetts at Amherst.

33. Sutton, R. S., & Barto, A. G. (2018). *Reinforcement learning: An introduction.* Vol. 1. Cambridge, MA: MIT Press.

34. Sutton, R. S. (2009). *Deconstructing reinforcement learning.* Proceedings of the 26th International Conference on Machine Learning. Montreal, Quebec.

35. Niv, Y., Edlund, J. A., Dayan, P., & O'Doherty, J. P. (2012). Neural prediction errors reveal a risk-sensitive reinforcement learning process in the human brain. *Journal of Neuroscience, 32,* 551–562.

36. DeWitt, E. E. (2014). Neuroeconomics: A formal test of dopamine's role in reinforcement learning. *Current Biology, 24*(8), R321–4.

37. Botvinick, M. M., Niv, Y., & Barto, A. C. (2009). Hierarchically organized behavior and its neural foundations: A reinforcement learning perspective. *Cognition, 113*(3), 262–280.

38. Moriarty, D. E., Schultz, A. C., & Grefenstette, J. J. (1999). Evolutionary algorithms for reinforcement learning. *Journal of Artificial Intelligence Research, 11,* 241–276.

39. Alija, J. A. (2010). *RoboCup soccer training: Using reinforcement learning to improve player skills.* Saarbrücken, Germany: LAP Lambert Academic.

40. Schultz, W. (2002). Getting formal with dopamine and reward. *Neuron, 36,* 241–263.

41. Khamassi, M., Lallée, S., Enel, P., Procyk, E., & Dominey, P. F. (2011). Robot cognitive control with a neurophysiologically inspired reinforcement learning model. *Frontiers in Neurorobotics, 5,* 1.

42. Wu, J., Xu, X., Zhange, P., & Liu, C. (2011). A novel multi-agent reinforcement learning approach for job scheduling in grid computing. *Future Generation Computer Systems, 27*(5), 430–439.

43. Mnih, V., Kavukcuoglu, K., Silver, D., Rusu, A. A., Veness, J., Bellemare, M. G., . . . Hassabis, D. (2015). Human-level control through deep reinforcement learning. *Nature, 518*(7540), 529–533.

44. Mustafa, K., Botteghi, N., Sirmacek, B., Poel, M., & Stramigioli, S. (2019). Towards continuous control for mobile robot navigation: A reinforcement learning and slam based approach. *ISPRS—International Archives of the Photogrammetry, Remote Sensing and Spatial Information Sciences, 4213,* 857–863.

45. Niv, Y. (2009). Reinforcement learning in the brain. *Journal of Mathematical Psychology, 53*(3), 139–154.

46. Schultz, W. (1998). Predictive reward signal of dopamine neurons. *Journal of Neurophysiology, 80,* 1–27.

47. Daw, N. D., Niv, Y., & Dayan, P. (2005). Uncertainty-based competition between prefrontal and dorsolateral striatal systems for behavioral control. *Nature Neuroscience, 8,* 1704–1711.

48. O'Doherty, J. P., Dayan, P., Friston, K., Critchley, H., & Dolan, R. J. (2003). Temporal difference models and reward-related learning in the human brain. *Neuron, 38*(2), 329–337.

49. D'Ardenne, K., McClure, S. M., Nystrom, L. E., & Cohen, J. D. (2008). BOLD responses reflecting dopaminergic signals in the human ventral tegmental area. *Science, 319*(5867), 1264–1267.

50. Zaghloul, K. A., Blanco, J. A., Weidemann, C. T., McGill, K., Jaggi, J. L., Baltuch, G. H., & Kahana, M .J. (2009). Human substantia nigra neurons encode unexpected financial rewards. *Science, 323*(5920), 1496–1499.

51. Montague, P. R., Hyman, S. E., & Cohen, J. D. (2004). Computational roles for dopamine in behavioural control. *Nature, 431,* 760–767.

52. Rescorla, R. A., & Wagner, A. R. (1972). A theory of Pavlovian conditioning: Variations in the effectiveness of reinforcement and nonreinforcement. In A. H. Black & W. F. Prokasy (Eds.), *Classical conditioning II: Current research and theory* (pp. 64–99). New York, NY: Appleton-Century-Crofts.

53. Schultz, W. (2000). Multiple reward signals in the brain. *Nature Reviews Neuroscience, 1,* 199–206.

54. Waelti, P., Dickinson, A., & Schultz, W. (2001). Dopamine responses comply with basic assumptions of formal learning theory. *Nature, 412,* 43–48.

55. Singh, S., Lewis, R. L., Barto, A. G., & Sorg, J. (2010). Intrinsically motivated reinforcement learning: An evolutionary perspective. *IEEE Transactions on Autonomous Mental Development, 2,* 70–82.

56. Ajzen, I., & Fishbein, M. (1980). *Understanding attitudes and predicting social behavior.* Englewood Cliffs, NJ: Prentice Hall.

57. Ulam, P., & Balch, T. (2003, December). *Niche selection for foraging tasks in multirobot teams using reinforcement learning.* Paper presented at the 2nd International Workshop on the Mathematics and Algorithms of Social Insects. Atlanta, GA.

58. Carver, C. S., & Scheier, M. R. (1998). *On the self-regulation of behavior.* New York, NY: Cambridge University Press.

59. Martin, G., & Pear, J. (2007). *Behavior modification: What it is and how to do it* (8th ed.). Upper Saddle River, NJ: Pearson Prentice Hall.

60. Prochaska, J., & DiClemente, C. (1983). Stages and processes of self-change of smoking: Toward an integrative model of change. *Journal of Consulting and Clinical Psychology, 51,* 390–395.

61. Rao, R. P., & Ballard, D. H. (1999). Predictive coding in the visual cortex: A functional interpretation of some extra-classical receptive-field effects. *Nature Neuroscience, 2*(1), 79–87.

62. Montague, P. R., & Berns, G. S. (2002). Neural economics and the biological substrates of valuation. *Neuron, 36,* 265–284.

63. Friston, K. (2010). Perception: A free-energy formulation. *International Perspectives on Psychological Science: Cognition and Neuropsychology, 1,* 49.

64. Shadmehr, R., Smith, M. A., & Krakauer, J. W. (2010). Error correction, sensory prediction, and adaptation in motor control. *Annual Review of Neuroscience, 33,* 89–108.

65. Doya, K. (2007). *Bayesian brain: Probabilistic approaches to neural coding.* Cambridge, MA: MIT Press.

66. Bubic, A., Von Cramon, D. Y., & Schubotz, R. I. (2010). Prediction, cognition and the brain. *Frontiers in Human Neuroscience, 4,* 25.

67. Bar, M. (2007). The proactive brain: Using analogies and associations to generate predictions. *Trends in Cognitive Science, 11*(7), 280–289.

68. Friston, K. J., & Stephan, K. E. (2007). Free-energy and the brain. *Synthese, 159*(3), 417–458.

69. Redish, A. D. (2013). *The mind within the brain: How we make decisions and how those decisions go wrong.* Oxford, England: Oxford University Press.

70. Hawkins, J., & Blakeslee, S. (2004). *On intelligence: How a new understanding of the brain will lead to the creation of truly intelligent machines.* New York, NY: Henry Holt.

71. Roesch, M. R., Esber, G. R. Li, J., Daw, N. D., & Schoenbaum, G. (2012). Surprise! Neural correlates of Pearce-Hall and Rescorla-Wagner coexist within the brain. *European Journal of Neuroscience, 35*(7), 1190–1200.

72. Morrison, V., & Bennett, P. (2009). *An introduction to health psychology* (2nd ed.). Harlow, England: Pearson Education.

73. Flay, B., & Petraitis, J. (1994). The theory of triadic influence. *Advances in Medical Sociology, 4*, 19–44.

74. Lockwood, T. (2009). *Design thinking: Integrating innovation, customer experience, and brand value.* New York, NY: Allworth Press.

75. Hohwy, J. (2012). Attention and conscious perception in the hypothesis testing brain. *Frontiers in Psychology, 3*, 96.

76. Biran, A., Schmidt, W.-P., Wright, R., Jones, T., Seshadri, M., Isaac, P., . . . Curtis, V. (2009). The effect of a soap promotion and hygiene education campaign on handwashing behaviour in rural India: A cluster randomised trial. *Tropical Medicine & International Health, 14*(10), 1303–1314.

77. Barker, R. G. (1968). *Ecological psychology: Concepts and methods for studying the environment of human behavior.* Palo Alto, CA: Stanford University Press.

78. Gautam, O. P., Schmidt, W. P., Cairncross, S., Cavill, S., & Curtis. V. (2017). Trial of a novel intervention to improve multiple food hygiene behaviors in Nepal. *The American Journal of Tropical Medicine and Hygiene, 96*(6), 1415–1426.

79. Schoggen, P. (1989). *Behaviour settings: A revision and extension of Roger G. Barker's ecological psychology.* Stanford, CA: Stanford University Press.

80. Barker, R. G. (1987). Prospecting in environmental psychology. In D. Stokols & I. Altman (Eds.), *Handbook of environmental psychology* (Vol. 2, pp. 1413–1432). New York, NY: Wiley.

81. Whitelaw, S., Baxendale, A., Bryce, C., MacHardy, L., Young, I., & Witney, E. (2001). "Settings" based health promotion: A review. *Health Promotion International, 16*, 339–353.

82. Dooris, M. (2009). Holistic and sustainable health improvement: The contribution of the settings-based approach to health promotion. *Perspectives in Public Health, 129*(1), 29–36.

83. Orbell, S., & Sheeran, P. (2002). Changing health behaviours: The role of implementation intentions. In D. R. Rutter & L. Quine (Eds.), *Changing health behaviour: Intervention and research with social cognition models* (pp. 123–137). Buckingham, England: Open University Press.

84. Gollwitzer, P. M., & Sheeran, P. (2006). Implementation intentions and goal achievement: A meta-analysis of effects and processes. *Advances in Experimental Social Psychology, 38*, 249–268.

85. McDaniel, M. A., & Einstein, G. O. (2007). *Prospective memory: An overview and synthesis of an emerging field.* Thousand Oaks, CA: SAGE.

86. Chasteen, A. L., Park, D. C., & Schwarz, N. (2001). Implementation intentions and facilitation of prospective memory. *Psychological Science, 12*, 457–461.

87. Tobias, R. (2009). Changing behavior by memory aids: A social psychological model of prospective memory and habit development tested with dynamic field data. *Psychological Review, 116*, 408–438.

88. Lang, A. (2000). The limited capacity model of mediated message processing. *Journal of Communication, 50*(1), 46–70.

89. Kovach, C. K., Daw, N. D., Rudrauf, D., Tranel, D., O'Doherty, J. P., & Adolph, R. (2012). Anterior prefrontal cortex contributes to action selection through tracking of recent reward trends. *The Journal of Neuroscience, 32*(25), 8434–8442.

90. Gilmor, T. M. (1978). Locus of control as a mediator of adaptive behaviour in children and adolescents. *Canadian Psychological Review/Psychologie canadienne, 19*(1), 1.

91. Moran, J. M., Jolly, E., & Mitchell, J. P. (2014). Spontaneous mentalizing predicts the fundamental attribution error. *Journal of Cognitive Neuroscience, 26*(3), 569–576.

92. Johnson, D. D., Blumstein, D. T., Fowler, J. H., & Haselton, M. G. (2013). The evolution of error: Error management, cognitive constraints, and adaptive decision-making biases. *Trends in Ecology & Evolution, 28*(8), 474–481.

93. Kramer, R. (1994). The sinister attribution error: Paranoid cognition and collective distrust in organizations. *Motivation and Emotion, 18*(2), 199–230.

94. Andrews, P. W. (2001). The psychology of social chess and the evolution of attribution mechanisms: Explaining the fundamental attribution error. *Evolution and Human Behavior, 22*(1), 11–29.

95. Aunger, R., & Curtis, V. (2014). The Evo-Eco approach to behaviour change. In D. W. Lawson & M. Gibson (Eds.), *Applied evolutionary anthropology* (pp. 271–295). London., England: Springer.

96. Aunger, R., & Curtis, V. (2015). *Gaining control: How human behaviour evolved.* Oxford, England: Oxford University Press.

97. Constant, A., Ramstead, M. J. D., Veissière, S. P. L., Campbell, J. O., &. Friston, K. (2018). A variational approach to niche construction. *Journal of the Royal Society: Interface, 15*(141).

98. Simon, H. (1974). How big is a chunk? *Science, 183,* 482–488.

99. Terrace, H. S. (2001). Chunking and serially organized behavior in pigeons, monkeys and humans. In R. G. Cook (Ed.), *Avian visual cognition.* Medford, MA: Comparative Cognition Press.

100. Ostlund, S. B., Winterbauer, N. E., & Balleine, B. W. (2009). Evidence of action sequence chunking in goal-directed instrumental conditioning and its dependence on the dorsomedial prefrontal cortex. *The Journal of Neuroscience, 29,* 8280–8287.

101. Schoggen, M., Barker, L. S., & Barker, R. G. (1963). Structure of the behavior of American and English children. In R. G. Barker (Ed.), *The stream of behavior: Explorations of its structure & content* (pp. 160–168). East Norwalk, CT: Appleton-Century-Crofts.

102. Schank, R., & Abelson, R. (1977). *Scripts, plans, goals and understanding: An inquiry into human knowledge structures.* Hillsdale, NJ: Erlbaum.

103. Zacks, J. M., & Tversky, B. (2001). Event structure in perception and conception. *Psychological Bulletin, 127,* 3–21.

104. Pinker, S. (1994). *The language instinct.* London, England: Allen Lane.

105. Barto, A. G., & Mahadevan, S. (2003). Recent advances in hierarchical reinforcement learning. *Discrete Event Dynamic Systems, 13*(4), 341–379.

106. Botvinick, M. M. (2008). Hierarchical models of behavior and prefrontal function. *Trends in Cognitive Science, 12*(5), 201–208.

107. Sutton, R. S., Precup, D., & Singh, S. (1999). Between MDPs and semi-MDPs: A framework for temporal abstraction in reinforcement learning. *Artificial Intelligence, 112,* 181–211.

108. Badre, D., & Frank, M. (2012). Mechanisms of hierarchical reinforcement learning in cortico-striatal circuits 2: Evidence from fMRI. *Cerebral Cortex, 22*(3), 527–536.

109. Dayan, P., & Niv, Y. (2008). Reinforcement learning: The good, the bad and the ugly. *Current Opinion in Neurobiology, 18*(2), 185–196.

110. Ribas-Fernandes, J., Solway, A., Diuk, C., McGuire, J. T., Barto, A. G., Niv, Y., & Botvinick, M. M. (2011). A neural signature of hierarchical reinforcement learning. *Neuron, 71,* 370–379.

111. Dietterich, T. G. (2000). Hierarchical reinforcement learning with the MAXQ value function decomposition. *Journal of Artificial Intelligence Research, 13,* 227–303.

112. Parr, R., & Russell, S. (1998). Reinforcement learning with hierarchies of machines. *Advances in Neural Information Processing Systems, 10,* 1043–1049.

113. Hebb, D. O. (1949). *The organization of behavior.* New York, NY: John Wiley.

114. Swanson, L. W. (2003). *Brain architecture: Understanding the basic plan.* Oxford, England: Oxford University Press.

115. Hawkins, J., & Blakeslee, S. (2004). *On intelligence.* New York, NY: Henry Holt.

116. Friston, K. (2009). The free-energy principle: A rough guide to the brain? *Trends in Cognitive Sciences, 13*(7), 293–301.

117. Hohwy, J. (2013). *The predictive mind.* Oxford, England: Oxford University Press.

118. Pearce, J. M., & Hall, G. (1980). A model for Pavlovian learning: Variations in the effectiveness of conditioned but not of unconditioned stimuli. *Psychological Review, 87*(6), 532.

119. Churchland, P., & Sejnowski, T. J. (1992). *The computational brain.* Boston, MA: MIT Press.

120. Llinas, R. (2002). *I of the vortex: From neurons to self.* Cambridge, MA: MIT Press.

121. Rolls, E. T. (1999). *The brain and emotion.* Oxford, England: Oxford University Press.

122. Daw, N. D., Niv, Y., & Dayan, P. (2005). Actions, policies, values and the basal ganglia. In E. Bezard (Ed.), *Recent breakthroughs in basal ganglia research* (pp. 91–106). New York, NY: Nova Science.

123. Daw, N. D., Gershman, S. J., Seymour, B., Dayan, P., & Dolan, R. J. (2011). Model-based influences on humans' choices and striatal prediction errors. *Neuron, 69*(6), 1204–1215.

124. Dayan, P., Niva, Y., Seymour, B., & Dawa, N. D. (2006). The misbehavior of value and the discipline of the will. *Neural Networks, 19*(8), 1153–1160.

125. Wunderlich, K., Dayan, P., & Dolan, R. J. (2012). Mapping value based planning and extensively trained choice in the human brain. *Nature Neuroscience,15*(5), 786–791.

126. Pavlov, I. P. (1927). *Conditioned reflexes: An investigation of the physiological activity of the cerebral cortex . . .* Translated and edited by G. V. Anrep. Oxford, England: Oxford University Press.

127. Abramson, C. (1994). *A primer of invertebrate learning: The behavioral perspective.* Washington, DC: American Psychological Association.

128. Krasne, F. B., & Glanzman, D. L. (1995). What we can learn from invertebrate learning. *Annual Review of Psychology, 46,* 585–624.

129. Mackintosh, N. J. (1985). *Conditioning and associative learning.* Oxford, England: Oxford University Press.

130. Staddon, J. E. R. (2003). *Adaptive behavior and learning* (2nd electronic ed.). Duke, NC: Duke University. http://psychandneuro.duke.edu/research/labs/staddon-lab.

131. Garcia, J., & Koelling, R. (1966). Relation of cue to consequence in avoidance learning. *Psychonomic Science, 4,* 123—124.

132. Neal, D. T., Lally, P., Wood, W., & Wu, M. (2009). *Do habits depend on goals? Perceived versus actual role of goals in habit performance.* Manuscript under review.

133. Ouellette, J., & Wood, W. (1998). Habit and intention in everyday life: The multiple processes by which past behavior predicts future behavior. *Psychological Bulletin, 124,* 54–74.

134. Willis, W. D. (1985). *The pain system: The neural basis of nociceptive transmission in the mammalian nervous system*. Basel, Switzerland: Kragel.

135. Streidter, G. F. (2005). *The principles of brain evolution*. Sunderland, MA: Sinauer Associates.

136. Northcutt, R. G., & Kaas, J. H. (1995). The emergence and evolution of mammalian neocortex. *Trends in the Neurosciences, 18*, 373–379.

137. Butler, A. B. (2001). Brain evolution and comparative neuroanatomy. In *Encyclopedia of the life sciences* (pp. 1–8). London, England: Macmillan.

138. Balleine, B. W., & Dickinson, A. (1998). Goal-directed instrumental action: Contingency and incentive learning and their cortical substrates. *Neuropharmacology, 37*, 407–419.

139. Berridge, K. C., & Robinson, T. E. (2003). Parsing reward. *Trends in Neurosciences, 26*, 507–513.

140. Burke, A., Heuer, F., & Reisberg, D. (1992). Remembering emotional events. *Memory & Cognition, 20*, 277–290.

141. Kensinger, E., & Corkin, S. (2004). Two routes to emotional memory: Distinct neural processes for valence and arousal. *Proceedings of the National Academy of Sciences of the United States of America, 101*, 3310–3315.

142. Valentin, V. V., Dickinson, A., & O'Doherty, J. P. (2007). Determining the neural substrates of goal-directed learning in the human brain. *The Journal of Neuroscience, 27*(15), 4019–4026.

143. Tolman, E. (1948). Cognitive maps in rats and men. *Psychology Review, 55*, 189–208.

144. Kopp, B. (2012). A simple hypothesis of executive function. *Frontiers of Human Neuroscience, 6*, 159.

145. Baars, B. (1997). *In the theater of consciousness: The workspace of the mind*. New York, NY: Oxford University Press.

146. Tulving, E. (1985). How many memory systems are there? *American Psychologist, 40*, 385–398.

147. Eichenbaum, H. (2000). Declarative memory. *Nature Reviews Neuroscience, 1*, 41–50.

148. Rolls, E. T. (2005). *Emotion explained*. Oxford, England: Oxford University Press.

149. Talmi, D., Seymour, B., Dayan, P., & Dolan, R. J. (2008). Human pavlovian–instrumental transfer. *The Journal of Neuroscience, 28*(2), 360–368.

150. Daw, N. D., & Shohamy, D. (2008). The cognitive neuroscience of motivation and learning. *Social Cognition, 26*(5), 593–620.

151. Dickinson, A., & Balleine, B. (2002). The role of learning in the operation of motivational systems. In H. Pashler & R. Gallistel (Eds.), *Stevens' handbook of experimental psychology* (3rd ed., pp. 497–534). New York.: Wiley.

152. Balleine, B. W., & O'Dohety, J. P. (2010). Human and rodent homologies in action control: Corticostriatal determinants of goal-directed and habitual action. *Neuropsychopharmacology, 35*, 48–69.

153. Dickinson, A. (1985). Actions and habits: The development of behavioral autonomy. *Philosophical Transactions of the Royal Society of London B: Biological Science, 308*, 67–78.

154. Everitt, B. J., & Robbins, T. W. (2005). Neural systems of reinforcement for drug addiction: From actions to habits to compulsion. *Nature Neuroscience, 8*, 1481–1489.

155. Yin, H. H., & Knowlton, B. J. (2006). The role of the basal ganglia in habit formation. *Nature Neuroscience, 7,* 464–476.

156. Pasupathy, A., & Miller, E. K. (2005). Different time courses of learning-related activity in the prefrontal cortex and striatum. *Nature, 433,* 873–876.

157. Thorndike, E. L. (1901). *Animal intelligence: An experimental study of the associative processes in animals.* Psychological Review Monograph Supplement 2. Lancaster, PA: Macmillan.

158. Poldrack, R. A., Sabb, F. W., Foerde, K., Tom, S. M., Asarnow, R. F., Bookheimer, S. Y., & Knowlton, B. J. (2005). The neural correlates of motor skill automaticity. *Journal of Neuroscience, 25,* 5356–5364.

159. Breland, K., & Breland, M. (1961). The misbehavior of organisms. *American Psychologist, 16*(11), 681.

160. Squire, L. R. (2004). Memory systems of the brain: A brief history and current perspective. *Neurobiology of Learning and Memory, 82,* 171–177.

161. Bullemer, P., Nissen, M., & Willingham, D. B. (1989). On the development of procedural knowledge. *Journal of Experimental Psychology: Learning, Memory and Cognition, 15,* 1047–1060.

162. Neal, D. T., Wood, W., & Quinn, J. M. (2006). Habits—A repeat performance. *Current Directions in Psychological Science, 15,* 198–202.

163. Berridge, K. C. (2009). "Liking" and "wanting" food rewards: Brain substrates and roles in eating disorders. *Physiology & Behavior, 97*(5), 537–550.

164. Aunger, R., & Curtis, V. (2008). Kinds of behaviour. *Biology and Philosophy, 23*(3), 317–345.

165. Aunger, R., & Curtis, V. (2013). The anatomy of motivation: An evolutionary ecological approach. *Biological Theory, 8,* 49–63.

166. Wilson, T. (2004). *Strangers to ourselves: Discovering the adaptive unconscious.* Cambridge MA: Belknap.

167. Kahneman, D. (2011). *Thinking, fast and slow.* New York, NY: Macmillan.

168. Biran, A., Schmidt, W.-P., Varadharajan, K. S., Rajaraman, D., Kumar, R., Greenland, K., . . . Curtis, V. (2014). Effect of a behaviour-change intervention on handwashing with soap in India (SuperAmma): A cluster-randomised trial. *The Lancet Global Health, 2*(3), e145–e154.

169. Aunger, R., Coombes, Y., Curtis, V., Mosler, H., & Travaskis, H. (2014). Changing WASH behaviour. In P. Cross & Y. Coombes (Eds.), *Sanitation and hygiene in Africa: Where do we stand? Analysis from the AfricaSan Conference, Kigali, Rwanda* (pp. 45–52). London, England: IWA Publishing.

170. Khamassi, M., & Humphries, M. D. (2012). Integrating cortico-limbic-basal ganglia architectures for learning model-based and model-free navigation strategies. *Frontiers in Behavioral Neuroscience, 6,* 79.

171. Dayan, P., & Berridge, K. C. (2014). Model-based and model-free Pavlovian reward learning: Revaluation, revision, and *revelation. Cognitive, Affective, & Behavioral Neuroscience, 14*(2), 473–492.

172. Ludvig, E. A., Sutton, R. S., & Kehoe, E. J. (2012). Evaluating the TD model of classical conditioning. *Learning & Behavior, 40*(3), 305–319.

173. Johnson, A., & Redish, A. D. (2005). Hippocampal replay contributes to within session learning in a temporal difference reinforcement learning model. *Neural Networks, 18*(9), 1163–1171.

174. Lee, S. W., Shimojo, S., & O'Doherty, J. P. (2014). Neural computations underlying arbitration between model-based and model-free learning. *Neuron, 81*(3), 687–699.

175. Aunger, R. (2010). What's special about human technology? *Cambridge Journal of Economics, 34,* 115–123.

176. Fleck, J. (2000). The artefact-activity couple: The co-evolution of artefacts, knowledge and organization in technological innovation. In J. Ziman (Ed.), *Technological innovation as an evolutionary process.* Cambridge, England: Cambridge University Press.

177. Ambrose, S. H. (2001). Paleolithic technology and human evolution. *Science, 291,* 1748–1753.

178. Grant, P. R., & Grant, B. R. (2002). Unpredictable evolution in a 30-year study of Darwin's finches. *Science, 296,* 707–711.

179. Michalak, J., Troje, N. F., Fischer, J., Vollmar, P., Heidenreich, T., & Schulte, D. (2009). Embodiment of sadness and depression—gait patterns associated with dysphoric mood. *Psychosomatic Medicine, 71*(5), 580–587.

180. Glenberg, A. M. (2010). Embodiment as a unifying perspective for psychology. *Wiley Interdisciplinary Reviews: Cognitive Science, 1*(4), 586–596.

181. Gallagher, S. (2005). *How the body shapes the mind.* Cambridge, England: Cambridge University Press.

182. James, W. (1884). What is an emotion? *Mind, 19,* 188–204.

183. Hull, C. L. (1943). *Principles of behavior: An introduction to behavior theory.* New York, NY: Appleton-Century.

184. Yerkes, R. M., & Dodson, J. D. (1908). The relation of strength of stimulus to rapidity of habit-formation. *Journal of Comparative Neurology and Psychology, 18,* 459–482.

185. Gershman, S. J., Pesaran, B., & Daw, N. D. (2009). Human reinforcement learning subdivides structured action spaces by learning effector-specific values. *The Journal of Neuroscience, 29*(43), 13524–13531.

186. Lakoff, G., & Johnson, M. (1999). *Philosophy in the flesh: The embodied mind and its challenge to Western thought.* New York, NY: Basic Books.

187. Varela, F., Thompson, E., & Rosch, E. (1991). *The embodied mind.* Cambridge, MA: MIT Press.

188. Miles, L. K., Nind, L. K., & Macrae, C. N. (2010). Moving through time. *Psychological Science, 21*(2), 222–223.

189. Cole, S., Balcetis, E., & Dunning, D. (2013). Affective signals of threat increase perceived proximity. *Psychological Science, 24*(1), 34–40.

190. Friston, K. (2011). Embodied inference: Or "I think therefore I am, if I am what I think." In W. Tschacher & C. Bergomi (Eds.), *The implications of embodiment: Cognition and communication* (pp. 89–125). Exeter, England: Imprint Academic.

191. Funder, D. C., & Guillaume, E. (2012). The person-situation debate and the assessment of situations. *Japanese Journal of Personality*/パーソナリティ研究, *21*(1), 1–11.

192. Rauthmann, J. F., Sherman, R. A., & Funder, D. C. (2015). Principles of situation research: Towards a better understanding of psychological situations. *European Journal of Personality, 29*(3), 363–381.

193. Kristjánsson, K. (2012). Situationism and the concept of a situation. *European Journal of Philosophy, 20*(Suppl. 1), E52–E72.

194. Tuomela, R. (2013). *Social ontology: Collective intentionality and group agents.* Oxford, England: Oxford University Press.

195. Caporael, L. R. (2003). Repeated assembly: Prospects for saying what we mean. In S. Scher & F. Rauscher (Eds.), *Evolutionary psychology: Alternative approaches* (pp. 71–90). New York, NY: Kluwer.

196. Krebs, J. R., & Dawkins, R. (1978). Animal signals: Mind reading and manipulation. In J. R. Krebs & N. B. Davies (Eds.), *Behaviour ecology: An evolutionary approach* (pp. 380–402). Sunderland, MA: Sinauer Associates.

197. Maynard Smith, J., & Harper, D. (2003). *Animal signals.* Oxford, England: Oxford University Press.

198. Lorenz, K. (1950). The comparative method in studying innate behaviour patterns. In J. F. Danielli & R. Brown (Eds.), *Physiological mechanisms in animal behaviour.* Cambridge, England: Cambridge University Press.

199. Serruya, D., & Eilam, D. (1996). Stereotypies, compulsions, and normal behavior in the context of motor routines in the rock hyrax *(Procavia capensis). Psychobiology, 24*(3), 235–246.

200. Barlow, G. (1977). Modal action patterns. In G. Barlow & T. Sebeok (Eds.), *How animals communicate* (pp. 98–134). Bloomington: Indiana University Press.

201. Young, M. (1988). *The metronomic society: Natural rhythms and human timetables.* Cambridge, MA: Harvard University Press.

202. Boyer, P., & Lienard, P. (2006). Why ritualized behavior? Precaution systems and action-parsing in developmental, pathological and cultural rituals. *Behavioral and Brain Sciences, 29,* 1–56.

203. Eilam, D., Zor, R., Szechtman, H., & Hermesh, H. (2006). Ritual, stereotypy and compulsive behavior in animals and humans. *Neuroscience and Biobehavioral Reviews, 30,* 456–471.

204. Barker, R. G., & Schoggen, P. (1973). *Qualities of community life: Methods of measuring environment and behavior applied to an American and an English town.* San Francisco, CA: Jossey-Bass.

205. Gibson, J. J. (1979). *The ecological approach to visual perception.* Boston, MA: Houghton Mifflin.

206. Goffman, E. (1971). *Relations in public: Microstudies of the public order.* New York, NY: Basic Books.

207. Goffman, E. (1959). *The presentation of self in everyday life.* Edinburgh, England: University of Edinburgh Social Sciences Research Centre.

208. Goffman, E. (1970). *Strategic interaction: An analysis of doubt and calculation in face-to-face, day-to-day dealings with one another.* Philadelphia: University of Pennsylvania Press.

209. Velleman, Y., Greenland, K., & Gautam, O. P. (2013). An opportunity not to be missed—immunisation as an entry point for hygiene promotion and diarrhoeal disease reduction in Nepal. *Journal of Water, Sanitation and Hygiene for Development, 3*(3), 459–466.

210. Hutchinson, G. E. (1957). Concluding remarks. *Cold Spring Harbor Symposia on Quantitative Biology, 22,* 415–427.

211. Povinelli, D. J. (2000). *Folk physics for apes: The chimpanzee's theory of how the world works.* Oxford, England: Oxford University Press.

212. Medin, D., & Atran, S. (1998). *Folk biology.* Cambridge, MA: MIT Press.

213. Ravenscroft, I. (2010). Folk psychology as a theory. In E. Zalta (Ed.), *Stanford encyclopedia of philosophy.* Stanford, CA: Stanford University.

214. Hirschfeld, L. (2001). On a folk theory of society: Children, evolution, and mental representations of social groups. *Personality and Social Psychology Review, 5,* 107–117.

215. Inagaki, K., & Hatano, G. (2006). Young children's conception of the biological world. *Current Directions in Psychological Science, 15*(4), 177–181.

216. Atran, S. (1998). Folk biology and the anthropology of science: Cognitive universals and cultural particulars. *Behavioral and Brain Sciences, 21*(4), 547–569.

217. Greif, M. L., Kemler Nelson, D. G., Keil, F. C., & Gutierrez, F. (2006). What do children want to know about animals and artifacts? Domain-specific requests for information. *Psychological Science, 17*(6), 455–459.

218. Aunger, R. (2010). Types of technology. *Technological Forecasting and Social Change, 77,* 762–782.

219. Mather, J. A., & Anderson, R. C. (1999). Exploration, play and habituation in *Octopus dofleini. Journal of Comparative Psychology, 113,* 333–338.

220. Kuba, M., Meisel, D. V., Byrne, R. A., Griebel, U., & Mather, J. A. (2003). Looking at play in *Octopus vulgaris. Berliner Paläobiol. Abh.,* 3, 163–169.

221. Grassé, P.-P. (1959). La Reconstruction du nid et les Coordinations Inter-Individuelles chez Bellicositermes Natalensis et Cubitermes sp. La théorie de la Stigmergie: essai d'interpretation du Comportement des Termites Constructeurs. *Insectes Sociaux, 6,* 41–81.

222. Orians, G., & Heerwagen, J. H. (1992). Evolved responses to landscapes. In J. H. Barkow, L. Cosmides, & J. Tooby (Eds.), *The adapted mind* (pp. 555–580). Oxford, England: Oxford University Press.

223. Mitani, J. C., Call, J., Kappeler, P. M., Palombit, R. A., & Silk, J. B. (Eds.). (2012). *The evolution of primate societies.* Chicago: University of Chicago Press.

224. Boehm, C. (1999). *Hierarchy in the forest: The evolution of egalitarian behavior.* Cambridge, MA: Harvard University Press.

225. Burghardt, G. M. (2005). *The genesis of animal play.* Cambridge, MA: MIT Press.

226. Vogel, I. (2012). *Review of the use of "theory of change" in international development.* London, England: UK Department for International Development.

227. Retolaza, I. (2011). Theory of change: A thinking and action approach to navigate in the complexity of social change processes. In *Hivos/UNDP/Democratic Dialogue.* Hivos/UNDP/Democratic Dialogue.

228. Stein, D., & Valters, C. (2012). *Understanding theory of change in international development.* London, England: Justice and Security Research Programme, London School of Economics.

229. Branson, R. K. (1975). *Interservice procedures for instructional systems development* (5 vols.). TRADOC Pam 350-30 NAVEDTRA 106A. Fort Monroe, VA: U.S. Army Training and Doctrine Command.

230. Anonymous. (2014). *2015 humanitarian needs overview guidance.* New York, NY: United Nations Office for the Coordination of Humanitarian Affairs.

231. Anonymous. (2008). *UNDG capacity assessment methodology user guide*. New York, NY: Capacity Development Group, United Nations Development Programme.

232. Gremba, J., & Myers, C. (1997). The IDEAL(SM) model: A practical guide for improvement. In *Bridge*. Software Engineering Institute, Carnegie Mellon.

233. Green, L., & Kreuter, M. (1991). *Health promotion planning* (2nd ed.). Mountain View, CA: Mayfield.

234. Curtis, V., Danquah, L. O., & Aunger, R. V. (2009). Planned, motivated and habitual hygiene behaviour: An eleven country review. *Health Education and Behavior, 4*, 655–667.

235. Griffiths, M., & Favin, M. (1999). Cultural tailoring in Indonesia's national nutrition improvement program. In R. A. Hahn (Ed.), *Anthropology in public health* (pp. 182–207). New York, NY: Oxford University Press.

236. Greenland, K., Chipungu, J., Chilengi, R., & Curtis, V. (2016). Theory-based formative research on oral rehydration salts and zinc use in Lusaka, Zambia. *BMC Public Health, 16*(1), 312.

237. Taplin, D. H., et al. (2013). *Theory of change*. New York, NY: ActKnowledge.

238. Young, D., Johnson, C. C., Steckler, A., Gittelsohn, J., Saunders, R. P., Saksvig, B. I., . . . McKenzie, T. L. (2006). Data to action: Using formative research to develop intervention programmes to increase physical activity in adolescent girls. *Health Education and Behaviour, 33*(1), 97–111.

239. Rothbauer, P. (2008). Triangulation. In L. Given (Ed.), *The SAGE encyclopedia of qualitative research methods* (pp. 892–894). London, England: SAGE.

240. Sawyer, K. (2008). *Group genius: The creative power of collaboration*. New York, NY: Basic Books.

241. Koestler, A. (1964). *The act of creation*. London, England: Hutchinsons.

242. Lakoff, G. (1987). Cognitive models and prototype theory. In U. Neisser (Ed.), *Concepts and conceptual development* (pp. 63–100). Cambridge, England: Cambridge University Press.

243. Fauconnier, G., & Turner, M. (2003). *The way we think: Conceptual blending and the mind's hidden complexities*. New York, NY: Basic Books.

244. Turner, M. (2014). *The origin of ideas: Blending, creativity, and the human spark*. Oxford, England: Oxford University Press.

245. Ozkan, B. E. (2004). *Autonomous Agent-based simulation of a model simulating the human air-threat assessment process*. Monterey, CA: Naval Postgraduate School.

246. Fauconnier, G., & Turner, M. (1998). Conceptual integration networks. *Cognitive Science, 22*(2), 133–187.

247. Coulson, S., & Fauconnier, G. (1999). Fake guns and stone lions: Conceptual blending and privative adjectives. In B. Fox, D. Jurafsky, & L. Michaelis (Eds.), *Cognition and function in language*. Palo Alto, CA: CSLI.

248. Michie, S., Wood, C. E., Johnston, M., Abraham, C., Francis, J. J., & Hardeman, W. (2015). Behaviour change techniques: The development and evaluation of a taxonomic method for reporting and describing behaviour change interventions (a suite of five studies involving consensus methods, randomised controlled trials and analysis of qualitative data). *Health Technology Assessment, 19*(99), 1–188.

249. Kok, G., Gottlieb, N. H., Peters, G.-J. Y., Dolan Mullen, P., Parcel, G. S., Ruiter, R. A. C., . . . Bartholomew, L. K. (2016). A taxonomy of behavior change methods: An intervention mapping approach. *Health Psychology Review, 10*(3), 297–312.

250. Crutzen, R., & Peters, G.-J. Y. (2018). Evolutionary learning processes as the foundation for behaviour change. *Health Psychology Review*, 12(1), 43–57.

251. Britton, B. K., & Pellegrini, A. D. (2014). *Narrative thought and narrative language*. New York, NY: Psychology Press.

252. Design Council. (2007). *Eleven lessons: Managing design in eleven global brands; A study of the design process*. London, England: Author.

253. Lewontin, R. C. (1970). The units of selection. *Annual Review of Ecology and Systematics*, 1, 1–18.

254. Watson, R. A., & Szathmary, E. (2016). How can evolution learn? *Trends in Ecology & Evolution*, 31(2), 147–157.

255. Hekler, E. B., Michie, S., Pavel, M., Rivera, D. E., Collins, L. M., Jimison, H. B., ... Spruijt-Metz, D. (2016). Advancing models and theories for digital behavior change interventions. *American Journal of Preventive Medicine*, 51(5), 825–832.

256. Nahum-Shani, I., Smith, S. N., Spring, B. J., Collins, L. M., Witkiewitz, K., Tewari, A., & Murphy, S. A. (2017). Just-in-time adaptive interventions (JITAIs) in mobile health: Key components and design principles for ongoing health behavior support. *Annals of Behavioral Medicine*, 52(6), 446–462.

257. Chandler, C. I., DiLiberto, D., Nayiga, S., Taaka, L., Nabirye, C., Kayendek, M., ... Staedke, S. G. (2013). The PROCESS study: A protocol to evaluate the implementation, mechanisms of effect and context of an intervention to enhance public health centres in Tororo, Uganda. *Implementation Science*, 8, 113.

258. Grant, A., Treweek, S., Dreischulte, T., Foy, R., & Guthrie, B. (2013). Process evaluations for cluster-randomised trials of complex interventions: A proposed framework for design and reporting. *Trials*, 14, 15.

259. De Silva, M. J., Breuer, E., Lee, L., Asher, L., Chowdhary, N., Lund, C., & Patel, V. (2014). Theory of change: A theory-driven approach to enhance the Medical Research Councils' framework for complex interventions. *Trials*, 15(1), 267.

260. Moore, G., Audrey, S., Barker, M., Bond, L., Bonell, C., Cooper, C., ... Barid, J. (2014). Process evaluation in complex public health intervention studies: The need for guidance. *Journal of Epidemiology & Community Health*, 68(2), 101–102.

261. Reynolds, J., DiLiberto, D., Mangham-Jefferies, L., Ansah, E. K., Lal, S., Mbakilwa, H., ... Chandler, C. I. R. (2014). The practice of "doing" evaluation: Lessons learned from nine complex intervention trials in action. *Implementation Science*, 9, 75.

262. Grossman, J., & Mackenzie, F. J. (2005). The randomized controlled trial: Gold standard, or merely standard? *Perspectives in Biology and Medicine*, 48(4), 516–534.

263. Cartwright, N., & Munro, E. (2010). The limitations of randomized controlled trials in predicting effectiveness. *Journal of Evaluation in Clinical Practice*, 16(2), 260–266.

264. Pawson, R. (2013). *The science of evaluation: A realist manifesto*. Thousand Oaks, CA: SAGE.

265. Victora, C. G., Habicht, J.-P., & Bryce, J. (2004). Evidence-based public health: Moving beyond randomized trials. *American Journal of Public Health*, 94(3), 400–405.

266. Richter, B., & Berger, M. (2000). Randomized controlled trials remain fundamental to clinical decision making in type II diabetes mellitus: A comment to the debate on randomized controlled trials. *Diabetologia*, 43(2), 254–258.

267. Melnyk, B. M., & Fineout-Overholt, E. (2011). *Evidence-based practice in nursing & healthcare: A guide to best practice.* Philadelphia, PA: Lippincott Williams & Wilkins.

268. Timmermans, S., & Mauck, A. (2005). The promises and pitfalls of evidence-based medicine. *Health Affairs, 24*(1), 18–28.

269. Curtis, V., Schmidt, W., Luby, S., Florez, R., Touré, O., & Biran, A. (2011). Hygiene: New hopes, new horizons. *The Lancet Infectious Diseases, 11*(4), 312–321.

270. Peikes, D. N., Moreno, L., & Orzol, S. M. (2008). Propensity score matching. *The American Statistician, 62*(3).

271. Kwasnicka, D., Dombrowski, S. U., White, M., & Sniehotta, F. (2016). Theoretical explanations for maintenance of behaviour change: A systematic review of behaviour theories. *Health Psychology Review, 10*(3), 277–296.

272. Yamey, G. (2011). Scaling up global health interventions: A proposed framework for success. *PLoS Medicine, 8*(6), e1001049.

273. Gillespie, S., Menon, P., & Kennedy, A. L. (2015). Scaling up impact on nutrition: What will it take? *Advances in Nutrition, 6*(4), 440–451.

274. Rajaramans, D., Varadharajan, K. S., Greenland, K., Curtis, V., Kumar, R., Schmidt, W.-P., . . . Biran, A. (2014). Implementing effective hygiene promotion: Lessons from the process evaluation of an intervention to promote handwashing with soap in rural India. *BMC Public Health, 19*(14), 1179.

275. Judah, G., de Witt Huberts, J., Drassal, A., & Aunger, R. (2017). The development and validation of a Real Time Location System to reliably monitor everyday activities in natural contexts. *PLoS One, 12*(2), e0171610.

Tables, figures and boxes are indicated by *t*, *f* and *b* following the page number

For the benefit of digital users, indexed terms that span two pages (e.g., 52–53) may, on occasion, appear on only one of those pages.

ABC (antecedent–behavior–consequence) model
  behavior as abstract in, 139n7
  feedback loops in, 9
ABCDE steps, 64–66, 110*f*, 124, 133–34
action selection, in BCD behavior challenge model, 27–29
adaptive programming, 114
affordance, 139n9
agent-based modeling, 129
Assessment step
  about, 64, 69
  behavior, 72–73
  behavior setting, 75–79
  body, 73–74
  brain, 73
  draft theory of change, 80
  environment (touchpoints), 74–75
  framing process, 70
  intervention, 79
  state of the world, 70–71
  SuperAmma Campaign example, 69, 72*b*, 73*b*, 74*b*, 75*b*, 76*b*
attribute ranking, 84

Barker, Roger, 24–25, 53–54*b*, 138n2, 139n9
Bayesian brain, 9
BCD behavior challenge model

basic problems of behavior change, 19–20
  causing revaluation, 21–23, 63–65
  central principle of, 29
  creating surprise, 20–21, 63–65
  enabling performance, 23–29, 63–65
  graphical representation of, 20*f*
  link to BCD theory of change, 139n1
  primary jobs of intervention, 19
BCD behavior determination model
  about, 31, 32*f*
  BCD theory
    behavior sequencing and reinforcement learning, 36*b*
    behavior settings, 52*b*
    evolution of behavioral control, 40*b*
    human motives, 45*b*, 45
  extended model
    approaches to behavior change, 48
    behavior, 35–36
    behavioral determinant checklist, 31, 33*t*
    behavior settings, 51–54
    body, 49–51
    brain, 38–48
    environment, 54–58
    graphical representation of, 32*f*
    RL models and levels of control, 48–49

BCD Manual, 61
BCD theory
    behavior sequencing and reinforcement
        learning, 36*b*
    behavior settings, 52*b*
    conceptual blending, 87*b*
    evolution of behavioral control, 40*b*
    human motives, 45*b*, 45
    link to BCD behavior challenge
        model, 139n1
    theory of change, 65*b*
behavior
    in BCD behavior determination
        model, 35–36
    definition of term, 35
behavioral control
    BCD behavior determination model
        hierarchical control architectures,
            36*b*, 36
        motivational-level control, 36, 41–44*b*
        planning and executive control, 47–48
        RL models and levels of control, 48–49
        three levels of control, 39–49
    evolution of, 40*b*
behavior centered design (BCD)
    ABCDE steps, 64–66, 133–34
    basic principle of, viii, 133
    benefits of, 132–33
    evolutionary framework of, 5
    extensions
        business development, 126–27
        marketing, 127–28
        policy-based change, 125–26
        self-help, 128–29
    future developments, 129–31
    observational, experimental, and
        intervention sciences, 131–32
    See also BCD behavior challenge
        model; BCD behavior
        determination model
behavior change
    BCD approach to
        benefits of, 17
        mismatch-specific solutions offered
            by, 16–18
    behaviors resistant to change, 9–10
    challenges of, 19–20

    concept of, 3–5
    impact of one behavior on another, 139n7
    introducing through interventions, 9–10
    need to update approach to, vii–viii
    See also BCD behavior challenge
        model; BCD behavior
        determination model
behavior change techniques (BCT),
    91–95, 92*t*
behavior demonstrations, 84
behavior sequencing, reinforcement
    learning and, 36*b*
behavior settings
    in BCD behavior challenge model,
        20*f*, 24–26
    in BCD behavior determination
        model, 51–54
    BCD theory and, 52*b*
    definition of term, 52*b*, 138n2
    repeated assembly concept, 139n8
    setting transfer problem, 26–27
behavior trials, 84
Behaviour-Centered Design website, 61
body, in BCD behavior determination
    model, 49–51
brain function
    in BCD behavior determination
        model, 38–48
        implications of three-level brain, 48
        motivated behavior, 39–45
        planning and executive control, 47–48
        reactive behavior, 39
        RL models and levels of
            control, 48–49
        three levels of control, 39–49
    error correction, 9
branding
    component analysis tool, 106*b*
    drawbacks of, 139n1
    importance of, 107
    increasing perception of value
        through, 17
Build step
    about, 64
    design process, 86–101
        component development, 90–91,
            92*t*, 97*b*

creative brief, 99–101
draft theory of change and campaign
      analysis, 95–96
gaining focus, 87–88
steps of, 86b
   formative research, 81–86
      far methods, 84
      hypothesis testing, 85
      in-between methods, 83–84
      near techniques, 82
      other methods, 85
   SuperAmma Campaign example, 82b,
      91b, 96b, 98b, 100b
business development, 126–27

campaign analysis, 95–101, 98b
co-creation, 82–83
component analysis, 106b
component development, 90–95, 92t, 97b
conceptual blending, 87b
Create step
   about, 64, 103b, 103
   creative process, 103–7
      component analysis tool, 106b
      managing a creative agency, 104b, 104
   field testing, 107–8
   report preparation, 108
   SuperAmma Campaign example, 108b,
      109b, 110b
creative agencies, managing, 104b, 104
creative brief, 99–101, 100b
credit assignment problem, 5
Crutzen, Rik, 93
curse of dimensionality, 36b
cybernetic cycles, 25

data collection, 81–86
   far methods, 84
   hypothesis testing, 85
   in-between methods, 83–84
   near techniques, 82
   other methods, 85
Delivery step
   about, 64–66, 111
   delivery strategies, 111–12
   monitoring, 112–15
   report preparation, 115

SuperAmma Campaign example,
      113b, 114b
demographic generations, technology
      adoption and, 10–13
design process, 86–101
   component development, 90–91, 92t, 97b
   creative brief, 99–101
   draft theory of change and campaign
      analysis, 95–96
   gaining focus, 87–88
   steps of, 86b
dimensionality, 36b
disability-adjusted life-years (DALYs),
      10–14, 11t
diseases of civilization, 10–14

emo-demos (emotional
      demonstrations), 92–93
environment, 54–58
   biological, 57t, 57–58
   physical, 56
   social, 58
error correction
   in brain function and learning, 9
   failures in, 10–15
Evaluation step
   dissemination, 122–24
   impact evaluation, 117–20
   overview of, 66, 117
   process evaluation, 120–22, 122b
   SuperAmma Campaign example, 119b,
      123b, 124b
evo-eco model, 138n1
evolutionary learning processes, 93
executive-level control, 36
external factors, precise definition of, 25

failure modes, 9
feedback loops, in normal course of
      learning, 4–10
fidelity
   campaign design analysis tool, 121
   message effectiveness and, 97b
   monitoring, 99
   process evaluation components list,
      114b, 122
   SuperAmma Campaign example, 112

field testing, 107–8, 108*b*
flexible programming, 114
focus group discussions, 84
follow-up, 124
formative research, 81–86
   far methods, 84
   hypothesis testing, 85
   in-between methods, 83–84
   near techniques, 82
   other methods, 85
free energy principle, 9

Gibson, J. J., 139n9
Goffman, Irving, 53–54*b*

hierarchical control architectures, 36*b*, 36
hypothesis testing, 85–86

impact evaluation, 117–20
interventions
   behavior change through, 9–10
   component development, 90–95, 92*t*, 97*b*
   evaluating, 117–24
   flexible or adaptive programming, 114
   primary jobs of, 19
interviews, 84

Just Checking monitoring system, 130

Kok, Gerjo, 93

learning process
   connection with BCD theory of
      change, 139n1
   factors resulting in public health
      problems, 137–38n5
   failures in, 10–15
   mismatch-specific solutions, 16–18
   normal course of, 5–10

marketing, 127–28
media monitoring specialists, 115
monitoring
   activity in home environments, 130–31
   programs outcomes, 112–15
motivation
   human motives in BCD theory, 45*b*, 45
   drives, 45–46

emotions, 46–47
   interests, 47
   lack of health benefits as, 138n1
   motivational-level control, 36, 41–44*b*
motive mapping, 84

nested intelligence, 9

on-site prototyping, 82

participant observation, 82
pathological learning, 13–15, 14*t*
perceptual error, 13
performance
   in BCD behavior challenge model, 20*f*,
      23–29, 63–65
   definition of term, 19
Peters, Gjalt-Jorn Ygram, 93
policy-based change, 125–26
prediction error
   in learning failures, 13–15
   in normal course of learning, 6
predictive brain hypothesis, error
   correction and, 9
proactive brain, 9
process evaluation, 120–22, 122*b*
program development
   BCD process model
      Assessment step, 69–80
      Build step, 81–101
      Create step, 103–10
      Delivery step, 111–15
      Evaluation step, 117–24
      graphical representation of, 64*f*
      overview of, 63–68
      SuperAmma Campaign example, 67*b*
      theory of change, 65*b*
   resources for, 61
proper domain motives, 23

QuietCare monitoring system, 130

randomized controlled trial (RCT), 117–18
real- time location system (RTLS), 130–31
reinforcement learning (RL)
   BCD RL model
      graphical representation of, 7*f*
      normal course of learning, 5–10

strength of, 137n1
effect of technological evolution
    on, 10–13
hierarchical, 36b, 36
modeling human learning behavior
    with, 5–10
separate steps of, 137n2
sources of error in, 13–15
See also BCD behavior
    determination model
report preparation
    Create step, 108
    Delivery step, 115
    Evaluation step, 122–23
revaluation
    in BCD behavior challenge model, 20f,
      21–23, 63–65
    definition of term, 19
reward mimic problem
    role in pathological learning, 13–14,
      14t, 15
    solutions to, 16
reward prediction errors, 13, 14t
role change, 25–26

scaling up programs, 123b
self-help, 128–29
self-regulation theory, 139n7
setting transfer problem, 26–27
side-effect mismatch
    cause of, 14–15
    solutions to, 16
social regulation theory, feedback
    loops in, 9

state prediction errors, 13–15, 14t
super-stimulating behaviors
    behaviors seen as health
      compromising, 137n3
    role in pathological learning, 14t, 14, 15
    solutions to, 16–17
surprise
    in BCD behavior challenge model, 20f,
      20–21, 63–65
    definition of term, 19

techno-generations, 10
technologies
    novel technologies as both cause and
      solution, 17
    rate of adoption, 3–5, 137n4
    role in lost DALYs, 10–15, 11t
temporal imbalance
    behaviors seen as health
      protective, 137n3
    definition of term, 15
    solutions to, 16–18
theory of change
    in Assessment step, 70, 80
    in Build step, 95–101, 96b
    causal links, 139n1
    concept of, 65b
transtheoretical model
    behavior as abstract, 139n7
    feedback loops in, 9

utility surprise, 13

video ethnography, 82